Clinical Nurse Specialist Toolkit

Melanie Duffy, MSN, RN, CCRN, CCNS is a Critical Care Clinical Nurse Specialist (CNS) at Pinnacle Health System, Harrisburg, Pennsylvania. She is a member of and certified by the American Association of Critical Care Nurses as a Critical Care Nurse (CCRN) and Critical Care Clinical Nurse Specialist (CCNS). Ms. Duffy is politically active and was instrumental in drafting and passing legislation for CNS Title Protection in Pennsylvania. She is an active member of the National Association of Clinical Nurse Specialists (NACNS) and the Legislative/Regulatory Committee of NACNS. Melanie is currently President-Elect of NACNS.

Susan Dresser, MSN, RN, CCRN, CNS-BC is a cardiovascular Clinical Nurse Specialist (CNS) at Deaconess Hospital, Oklahoma City, Oklahoma. She graduated from the University of North Carolina with a Bachelor of Science degree in Nursing and completed her Master of Science degree from Duke University as an Adult Critical Care CNS. Ms. Dresser is an active member of the American Association of Critical Care Nurses and has maintained certification as a Critical Care Nurse (CCRN) since 1980. She has held positions as a Cardiovascular and Critical Care CNS for the past 20 years. Ms. Dresser is adjunct faculty for the University of Central Oklahoma and the University of Oklahoma. She served as Director at Large on the Board of Directors for the National Association of Clinical Nurse Specialists (NACNS) and is the current Secretary of NACNS.

Janet S. Fulton, PhD, RN, ACNS-BC is the Program Coordinator, Adult Clinical Nurse Specialist Program, Indiana University School of Nursing, Indianapolis, Indiana. She is a past president of the National Association of Clinical Nurse Specialists (NACNS) and editor of *Clinical Nurse Specialist: The Journal for Advanced Nursing Practice.*

Clinical Nurse Specialist Toolkit

A Guide for the New Clinical Nurse Specialist

Melanie Duffy, MSN, RN, CCRN, CCNS
Susan Dresser, MSN, RN, CCRN, CNS–BC
Janet S. Fulton, PhD, RN, ACNS–BC

Editors

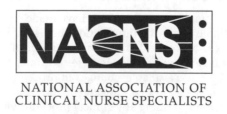

NATIONAL ASSOCIATION OF
CLINICAL NURSE SPECIALISTS

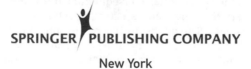

SPRINGER PUBLISHING COMPANY

New York

Springer Publishing Company, LLC
11 West 42nd Street
New York, NY 10036
www.springerpub.com

Acquisitions Editor: Margaret Zuccarini

Project Manager: Julia Rosen

Cover Designer: Steve Pisano

Composition: Apex CoVantage, LLC

Ebook ISBN: 978-0-8261-1836-3

09 10 11 12 13/ 5 4 3 2

Library of Congress Cataloging-in-Publication Data

Clinical nurse specialist toolkit : a guide for the new clinical nurse specialist / editors, Melanie Duffy, Susan Dresser, Janet S. Fulton.
    p. ; cm.
  Includes bibliographical references.
  ISBN 978-0-8261-1835-6 (alk. paper)
  1. Nurse practitioners. I. Duffy, Melanie. II. Dresser, Susan.
III. Fulton, Janet S.
  [DNLM: 1. Nurse Clinicians. 2. Nurse's Role. 3. Nursing Care.
WY 128 C6407 2009]

  RT82.8.C576 2009
  610.73092—dc22   2008050931

Printed in the United States of America by Hamilton Printing Company.

This book is lovingly dedicated to the memory of Kathryn Ann "Katie" Brush, clinical nurse specialist, humanitarian, and scholar whose deep devotion to those she served was marked with courage, compassion, and joy. She is loved, missed, and celebrated!

Contents

Contributors

Katie Brush, MS, RN, CCRN, CCNS, FCCM (Deceased)
Massachusetts General Hospital
Boston, Massachusetts

Ann M. Herbage Busch, MS, RN, CWOCN, ACNS-BC, CNS-PP
Portland Veterans Affairs Medical Center
Portland, Oregon

Vivian Donahue, MSN, RN, CCRN, ACNS-BC
Massachusetts General Hospital
Boston, Massachusetts

Patricia A. Foster, MS, RN, CMSRN, ACNS-BC
Chandler Regional Medical Center
Chandler, Arizona

Sharon D. Horner, PhD, RN, CNS
The University of Texas at Austin School of Nursing
Austin, Texas

Susan K. B. Jones, MS, RN, APN, CCNS-P, CCRN-P
INTEGRIS Health
Oklahoma City, Oklahoma

Deborah G. Klein, MSN, RN, CCRN, CS
Cleveland Clinic
Cleveland, Ohio

Cathy Lewis, MSN, RN
Mott Children's Hospital, University of Michigan Health System
Ann Arbor, Michigan

Melissa A. Lowder, MSN, RN, CCRN
St. Francis Hospital
Beech Grove, Indiana

Denise O'Brien, MSN, RN, ACNS-BC, CPAN, CAPA, FAAN
University of Michigan Health System
Ann Arbor, Michigan

Ginger S. Pierson, MSN, RN, CCRN, CNS
Hoag Memorial Hospital Presbyterian
Newport Beach, California

Jan Powers, PhD, RN, CCRN, CCNS, CNRN, CWCN, FCCM
St. Vincent Hospital
Indianapolis, Indiana

Christine Schulman, MS, RN, CNS, CCRN
Christine S. Schulman, LLC
Portland, Oregon

Patrick Schultz, MS, RN, ACNS-BC, CCRN
MeritCare Health System
Fargo, North Dakota

Susan Sendelbach, PhD, RN, CCNS, FAHA
Abbott Northwestern Hospital
Minneapolis, Minnesota

Mary A. Stahl, MSN, RN, ACNS-BC, CCNS-CMC, CCRN
Mid America Heart Institute, Saint Luke's Hospital
Kansas City, Missouri

Mary Fran Tracy, PhD, RN, CCNS, FAAN
University of Minnesota Medical Center, Fairview
Minneapolis, Minnesota

Ruth Van Gerpen, MS, RN, APRN-CNS, OCN
BryanLGH Medical Center
Lincoln, Nebraska

Kathleen M. Vollman, MSN, RN, CCNS, FCCM
ADVANCING NURSING, LLC
Northville, Michigan

Kathy Wright, MS, RN, CWOCN, CHRN, APRN
National Healing Corporation
Boca Raton, Florida

Ruthann B. Zafian, MSN, RN, MA, ACNS-BC, APRN
Hartford Hospital
Hartford, Connecticut

Preface

The idea for this book grew from a National Association of Clinical Nurse Specialists (NACNS) Board of Directors discussion on strategies to support the clinical nurse specialist (CNS) graduate transitioning into a first job as a CNS. Board members began sharing stories from their own transition periods, and it became evident that common themes ran through individual experiences. All board members present agreed that the wisdom about successful transition to the CNS role could be found in the narratives of those who made the journey. Hence, this book was conceived as a collection of practical tips and helpful information on selected topics written by experienced CNSs as advice to new CNSs.

This book is designed for a new CNS; however, it should be helpful for CNS students and all practicing CNSs looking for some new ideas. It is titled a *toolkit* because the focus is practical guidance for success around common challenges a CNS encounters. The authors shared lessons learned, personal insights, and proven strategies for succeeding in the CNS role from the perspective of experience. Chapter 1 begins with tips for negotiating a job, the final chapter contains some thoughts for a joyful career as a CNS, and in between readers will find advice on such topics as developing a job description, working with the boss, and obtaining certification. The chapters are concise, conversational, and practical by design.

As editors, we are indebted to the NACNS Board of Directors for their ideas and guidance. We thank our author contributors for sharing their expertise and personal stories. We are also indebted to the NACNS staff, especially Aleta Lazur, for their support, and to Margaret Zuccarini at Springer Publishing, for her guidance. Last, we say thank you to Christine Carson Filipovich, Chief Executive Officer, NACNS, for her help in making this book a reality and in making NACNS a beacon for CNSs everywhere.

Along the way, we lost a dear member of the board, Katie Brush. We are grateful to have Katie's chapter on prioritizing included in the book. In recognition of her service to NACNS as a board member and contributor to this project, the book is lovingly dedicated to Katie—gone too soon.

Melanie Duffy, MSN, RN, CCRN, CCNS
Susan Dresser, MSN, RN, CCRN, CNS-BC
Janet S. Fulton, PhD, RN, ACNS-BC

Getting
Started

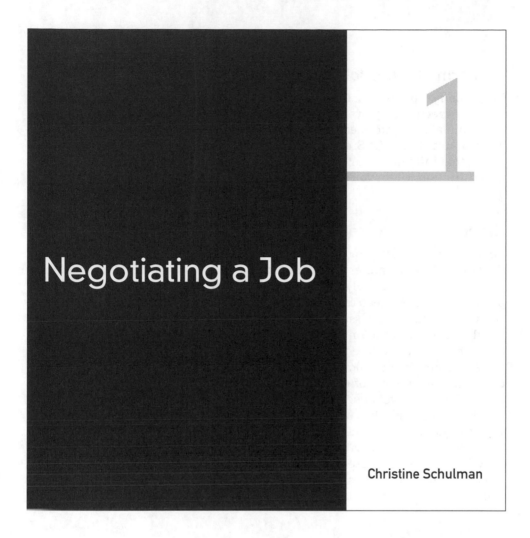

Negotiating a Job

Christine Schulman

The dream job for any clinical nurse specialist (CNS) is one that will be satisfying and challenging over time. Negotiating the fine details to make that happen is an ongoing process that starts at the time of hire and extends throughout the time you have the position. First things first, however: you must successfully navigate several phases of the job search process before you will negotiate the details of an exciting offer. Being clear on what you enjoy about your work, about the job you are being offered, and about what you personally need to be successful are essential for making an educated decision about your work. This chapter will first focus on reflecting about what you enjoy about being a CNS and then preparing for the job search. Next, it will provide suggestions for a powerful and insightful interview with a prospective employer, colleagues, and clients. Finally, key points to negotiate before accepting the job offer, along with specific items to address, will be discussed. A successful journey along these steps will help you identify and get the job that will create and sustain your professional enthusiasm over the long haul.

Preparing for the Job Search

Preparatory work for the interview is critical to making a good impression with your prospective employer as well as making sure you get the information you need to make an informed decision about the position. This includes thinking about your role as a CNS, developing your professional portfolio, identifying life issues that influence your ability to meet the job requirements, and researching the institution where you seek employment.

Reflect on Your Role as a CNS

Spend time preparing for the interview process by reflecting on your vision of the CNS role, your interests and talents, and your personal life issues that must be considered when applying for a position. Thinking about these things is important to ensure a good match between what you want and the actual job. Once you've identified these issues, be watchful for how they are addressed throughout the entire application process, beginning with the first interview until the time when you are offered the position.

Ask yourself the following questions: Why did I become a CNS? Which of the main components of the role (education and mentoring, quality improvement, protocol development, research) give me the most satisfaction? How do my skills align with the components of the role? Are my passions in alignment with the job requirements? What does the "perfect CNS day" look like? Answers to these questions provide structure for discussion during your interviews. Alignment of these important issues with what you've discovered about the job during the application process will influence your decision to accept or decline the job offer.

Prepare a Portfolio

You will be asked to describe your work experience. While a curriculum vitae (CV) or resume presents an excellent overview of your accomplishments, it doesn't reveal how you think, communicate, and accomplish work. A portfolio will help you show interviewers not just what you have accomplished but how you work. The "oral" portfolio consists of stories illustrating your experiences with communication, conflict management, prioritization, outcomes management, financial issues, and involvement with professional organizations. If you recently completed your graduate program, you will need to emphasize group and individual school projects. Have these examples fresh in your memory and well rehearsed so that they are concise and clearly illustrate your point. The "written" portfolio includes the hard copy evidence of your work. Depending on the position you're applying for, it should include some, if not all, of the following items:

- Published journal articles or book chapters, ideally regarding your area of expertise
- Printouts of research or quality improvement (QI) posters presented at professional conferences

- A handout from one of your best presentations
- A descriptive summary of a project you led, with outcome data (if not confidential)
- A protocol, policy, or procedure that you wrote
- An evaluation summary of a class you taught or course you coordinated

Identify Important Life Issues

Life issues are as important as your education and your experience in identifying whether you are able to meet the requirements of the job. These questions often address scheduling challenges (e.g., Do you need to arrive at work after 8:00 A.M.? Are you able to work the occasional evening and night shift? Do you need flexibility in your start and stop times due to child care or other transportation issues?). Think about how much time you can give the position; the reality of the CNS role is that there are always periods when you need to put in extra time to get work done. You need to know if your home responsibilities or personal energies are such that they cannot accommodate frequent overtime so that you don't accept a position where a usual workweek exceeds 50 hours.

Research the Prospective Employer

Resources in effective interviewing consistently state the importance of researching your potential workplace (Byham & Pickett, 1999; Pohly, n.d.; U.S. Department of Labor, 2005). How big is the institution? Is it an academic or a community facility? Is it a profit, nonprofit, or government-run entity? How many of its patients are Medicare patients? What are the Centers of Emphasis (in order to determine if its priorities are consistent with your areas of interest)? Is it a Magnet institution, or has it received other recognitions for excellence? What is its reputation in the nursing community? Is it unionized? Does it have a relationship with a university to support ongoing education of its employees? These questions identify the type of facility that will support your professional needs and interests over time. They will also help you develop questions you should ask during your interview to explore areas of interest or concern.

Preparing for the Interview

A full discussion of how to have an effective job interview is beyond the scope of this chapter; however, there are numerous excellent resources available to help you prepare for this event (Block & Petrus, 2004; Byham & Pickett, 1999; Fitzwater, 2001; Kessler, 2006; Powers, 2000; Welton, Morton, & Amig, 1998). The following discussion will focus on the elements that will help you identify key issues that usually surface during the final negotiations of a CNS position.

Develop responses to questions that are likely to be asked. Some questions will be simple and direct, such as: What is appealing to you about being a CNS? Are you able to work the night shift? What training do you have in data analysis? How do you communicate to others that you are stressed? Many employers use "behavioral interviews," which ask open-ended questions that allow you to describe real events and your role in them. The interviewer is looking for you to describe in detail your role in a particular event, project, or experience and what the outcome was (Fitzwater, 2001; Pohly, n.d.; Quintessential Careers, n.d.). Hearing about your past performance can help prospective employers predict your future performance in similar circumstances. Their objective is to identify your communication skills, how you prioritize work demands, your ability to resolve conflict, your clinical expertise, and your ability to navigate change. Use examples from school, internships, previous jobs, and volunteer work. Highlight special professional and personal accomplishments such as the money raised from a professional conference that you coordinated or the marathon that you finished within your expected time frame. Behavioral questions may also try to identify your response to negative situations and how you learn from them (Quintessential Careers, n.d.).

To prepare for behavior-based interviews, think about several examples where you demonstrated excellent performance in areas that the employer will be interested in: Clinical issues, team building, change management, and conflict resolution are commonly explored during interviews. You should also be prepared to describe situations that started out negatively but ended positively because you either made the best of the outcome or learned from that experience to behave differently the next time a similar situation arose. Make sure that your examples illustrate a variety of experiences from your work and professional life. Rehearse telling these stories so that you quickly get to the point and don't wander off topic; every story should have a clear beginning, middle, and end. Examples of questions likely to surface during your interview can be found in Table 1.1.

Use the STAR format to structure concise answers to behavioral questions (Quintessential Careers, n.d.).

- **Situation or Task:** Specifically describe the situation you were in or the task you needed to accomplish. Give enough detail for the interviewer to understand, but not so much that you wander off track or lose the attention of the interviewer.
- **Action:** Describe the action you took. Keep the focus of the story on your role and activities, even if describing a team project. Tell what you actually did do, not what you should have done.
- **Results:** Describe the outcome of the event. Were goals accomplished? What were the lessons learned?

An interview is a two-way street, so you must also plan to ask questions. Asking good questions will provide you with the information you need, and it will also demonstrate to your interviewer your critical thinking abilities and priorities (Block & Petrus, 2004; Career Consulting Corner, n.d.). This is not the time to ask about salary or work hours; this is the time to ask about relationships, priorities, and work processes at the institution in which you seek employment. Use the principles of behavioral interviews described above to encourage the interviewer to answer your questions with clear examples. Failure to take advantage of this opportunity could result in unpleasant surprises later and suggest to the interviewer that your level of interest and commitment to the job may be limited.

1.1 Behavioral Interview Questions for the CNS Candidate

- Describe how you implemented new research findings into practice at your institution.
- Tell about an incident where you formed and developed a team.
- Describe how you resolved a conflict with a supervisor, colleague, or client.
- Describe how you identified and managed a need within your institution.
- Give an example of when you had to share difficult feedback.
- Describe a quality or process improvement project that you coordinated.
- Tell about how you set and achieved a personal or professional goal.
- What is the most difficult project you have ever tackled and why? What was the outcome, and what did you learn from this experience?
- Tell about a time when you had to partner with someone whose work style was very different from yours.
- Give an example of a good (or bad) decision that you made and what you learned from that decision.
- Tell about a situation when you had to build consensus within a group of diverse people.
- Give an example of how you prioritized multiple demands. How did you manage your stress during this time?
- Describe a time when you had to communicate information or a practice change that was unpopular. How did you approach it, did you achieve buy-in, and what was the result?
- Describe a situation in which you had to support an administrative decision that you personally did not agree with. How did you do this? How did you reconcile this to yourself?
- Describe a project in which you had to maintain tight fiscal control. Did you accomplish your financial goals?
- How would you describe your management style? Give examples of when this has been helpful and when it has been a handicap.

All interviewers and interview panels should be asked to share their vision of the CNS role at the institution. They should also be asked to describe how past key projects have been prioritized, to identify initial needs that must be addressed, to describe the orientation plan and evaluation criteria, to clarify the reporting structure, to address the working style of the team, and to address a typical workday or workweek. Get clarification on who you will report to: Will this person be a nursing administrator, a hospital administrator, or a unit nurse manager? Ask to see the organizational structure of the facility and the nursing division so you can assess the power of nursing within that institution and the "political" climate. It is important to inquire about support for professional development opportunities (e.g., participation in professional organizations, writing for publication, presentations at national conferences, affiliations with industry).

Ask your prospective employer to clarify the scope of the job. Will you be responsible for a geographical clinical area or a specific patient population throughout the hospital (e.g., the sixth floor telemetry unit or all cardiology patients in the facility from Emergency Department admission to Cardiac Rehab)? Will you have responsibilities on several campuses within that hospital system? Will you be required to do direct patient care? Under what circumstances might this happen? Will you have responsibilities outside of your immediate clinical area (e.g., chair of the hospital-wide Pain committee, tracking and reporting central line and surgical site infection data within the system and nationally)? CNS and educator colleagues should be asked how they distribute the workload and communicate with one another. Ask for examples of how the supervisor advocated for them when there were multiple demands for CNS time. Similarities or differences in answers suggest the degree to which the team communicates and perceives the work environment.

Preparing to have an effective interview is of paramount importance. It provides the opportunity for a potential employer to learn about you and how you will contribute to the organization. No less important, however, the interview allows you to learn about that institution and determine whether it is a place in which you wish to work.

Negotiating the Job Offer

Once you have received a job offer, you are given another opportunity to fine-tune the position to sustain your professional interests without sacrificing important lifestyle issues. This is the time to negotiate the details to foster your professional success. You are in the driver's seat. You must clarify questions from your earlier interviews, further explore areas of concern or interest, and work out the details of financial compensation, benefits, and scheduling. Advocate for yourself, but show willingness to compromise to meet the needs of the organization while not sacrificing what is important to your long-term satisfaction and performance.

The first types of questions address the basic structure of your job. When do you start, relocation reimbursement, what your work schedule will be, and most importantly, salary and benefits. The last two items may be addressed by someone in human resources. Regardless of whom you speak with about salary, it is critical that you are familiar with the range of CNS salaries in your community. You need to know if the proposed compensation is comparable to what is available elsewhere in your region. Consider whether the salary, health care and vacation benefits, and support for professional advancement add up to a reasonable package compared with other options in your geographical area. For example, the salary might be slightly lower than the community standard, but this might be favorably balanced against something else that is particularly attractive to you, such as a tuition break if you wish to go back to school, flexible hours if you have children who have school transportation needs, or an option for a 4-day workweek rather than the traditional 5-day week. It all boils down to what is important to your professional and personal needs. CNSs are "jacks of all trades" who are invaluable to an institution and, therefore, should be compensated with time, money, and professional benefits to reflect this. If the sum of these benefits is substandard, then continue to negotiate or consider declining the offer.

It is important to clarify how your work will be assigned and prioritized. Work assignments coming from more than one person can result in conflict and unreasonable demands on your time. The ultimate result of this disorganization is that you will become frustrated, miss deadlines, and produce work that is not the quality that you prefer.

If you have not yet met with your immediate peer group, ask to do so now. Here you want to ask questions to help you ascertain the collegiality of the group. In other words, do they work and play well together? How do they distribute workload? How do they partner on projects? How do they cover for one another for illness, vacations, and holidays? Will you be part of a specific CNS group, and does participating in that group add to your responsibilities? Watch body language closely during this meeting. Is there laughter and a sense of cohesiveness in the group? Does anyone stand out as being different from the group or different from you, such that he or she might be difficult to work with? Much of the work of the CNS is relationship based, so it is important that your cohort be people you enjoy, you can work with, and you can learn from.

The next set of questions has to do with getting started in the role and ensuring that you will receive the technical support you need to do your work. They are listed in Table 1.2. Be leery of any promise to find you an office after you have started or situations where you are expected to share a computer. Hospitals frequently have limited office space. It could be months before you find a place to call "home," which could adversely impact your productivity. It may be necessary to negotiate your start date based on when your office is expected to be available. There is no need to be unrealistic regarding this issue, such as demanding a private office with a window! The ideal space for a CNS is one that places you either with your peer group or with the unit where you will be doing most of your work so that you are immediately accessible to the nursing staff, physicians, and your colleagues. Ask if it is permissible to work from home, especially when projects that require quiet time (e.g., writing an article) are under tight deadlines.

1.2 Negotiating the Fine Points of the Job Offer

- Will there be an office space established on the day that you start?
- Will there be a pager, phone, computer set up, and paperwork for computer and other passwords on the start date or reasonably soon thereafter?
- Is there clerical/administrative support when you need it?
- Will there be a parking space available? Will you have to pay for parking?
- How often will there be times when you are expected to leave the hospital mid-day such that having a car will be essential? Are there other transportation alternatives?
- Who will be your preceptor during orientation?
- How often should you meet with your supervisor during orientation?
- Who will give feedback during orientation and the first year?
- What are the priorities for the first 6 months? First year?

Another "red flag" is if there is no clerical or administrative support to help you with paperwork and routine office activities (e.g., processing course registrations, tallying course evaluations, data entry). While a CNS is certainly able to do these activities, your time and expertise is more appropriately spent on the clinical issues you were hired to work on. The institution you want to work for should have people in place so that you don't have to spend time doing secretarial work. Most CNSs will say it is oftentimes easier and quicker to do something themselves because they're thinking and creating while they type the document. That being said, there needs to be support for clerical tasks so that your energies can be focused on nursing concerns. Speaking with your potential peer group about the amount of administrative support will help you identify if this is an issue you need to consider before making your decision.

Thinking It Over

You have spent a lot of time and energy preparing for the interview that will lead to a job offer. In response to that offer, more issues have been explored, negotiated, and agreed upon. Finally, you have all of the information you need to make a smart decision about this professional opportunity. Your friends and colleagues will offer solicited and unsolicited advice, warnings, and encouragement. There is value in listening to their input, certainly, but it is more important that you listen to yourself and your internal dialogue. Is this a job that you want to do? Do you think it will be interesting? Will you like the patients, your colleagues, and the work you will be asked to do? Has there been good dialogue with the people you've met? Do you have a sense of how the job might evolve over time? Does it meet your professional goals? Does it put you in a good position to pursue your future professional development? Will the demands of the job work in concert with your responsibilities to your home and family? Does it feel like a "good fit"? Remember that every CNS job is unique and shaped by the facility's expectations of the role. Nonetheless, you still have major input into how the role plays out over time. Always look to the potential for how the role can be shaped and reshaped into what you want it to be.

While you are unable to read the future, you must make the decision with your head, your gut, and your heart about accepting this offer. Consider how this position meets your vision of the optimal CNS role and why you became a CNS. Review your experiences to date. Think about how those experiences, along with your passions and talents, align with the expectations of the job. Reflect upon the questions you were asked and ponder the answers to your questions during the interviews. Finally, consider how this job complements your personal life. Then, listen to your internal voice about what feels right . . . and decide!

References

Block, J., & Petrus, M. (2004). *Great answers! Great questions! To your job interview.* New York: McGraw-Hill.

Byham, W., & Pickett, D. (1999). *Landing the job you want.* New York: Three Rivers Press.

Career Consulting Corner. (n.d.). *Interview preparation Area 2*. Retrieved August 29, 2007, from http://www.careercc.com/interv3.shtml

Fitzwater, T. (2001). *Preparing for the behavior based interview*. Menlo Park, CA: Crisp Publications.

Kessler, R. (2006). *Competency based interviews: Master the tough new interview style*. Franklin Lakes, NJ: Career Press.

Pohly, Pam. (n.d.). *Successfully answer behavioral questions in your job interview*. Retrieved September 5, 2007, from http://www.pohly.com/interview-3.html

Powers, L. (2000). Anatomy of an interview. *AORN, 72*(4), 671–674.

Quintessential Careers. (n.d.). *STAR interviewing response technique for success in behavioral job interviews*. Retrieved September 5, 2007, from www.quintcareers.com/STAR_interviewing

U.S. Department of Labor. (2005, December 20). *Bureau of Labor statistics occupational outlook handbook. Job interview tips*. Retrieved September 5, 2007, from http://www.bls.gov/oco/oco20045.htm

Welton, R. H., Morton, P. G., & Amig, A. (1998). How to succeed in job interviewing. *Critical Care Nurse, 18*(1), 68–73.

2

Creating a Job Description

Kathleen M. Vollman,

Denise O'Brien,

and Cathy Lewis

The job description for clinical nurse specialist (CNS) is the foundation for practice of the role within an organization where the CNS is employed. A job description needs to be general enough to be inclusive of all variations of CNS practice but specific enough to serve as a roadmap for the essential role components to be actualized. In addition, a job description identifies the basic parameters for performance appraisal. If no job description exists, one should be created. Existing job descriptions should be reviewed and updated every several years.

Fundamentally a job description is an outline of the essential characteristics of the CNS role and includes minimal requirements for safe practice, such as education, certification, and experience. To achieve timely development or updating of a job description, focus on a consensus building process and use of evidence. The following is a list of suggested strategies to get started:

1. Use national standards as the foundation for core competencies of the CNS role.
2. Review the various types of CNS practice within the institution, such as unit based, program based, inpatient, or outpatient.

3. Create a team that includes representation from differing types of CNS practice and nursing administration, including both front-line manager and director level administrators.

Creating the Job Description

Using national standards as a foundation for the job description helps keep the job description within professional agreed upon boundaries. Standards help define the scope and practice of the CNS role regardless of specialty and ensure that entry level key characteristics and competencies are incorporated. Every job description should have an organizing framework. The National Association of Clinical Nurse Specialists (National Association of Clinical Nurse Specialists [NACNS], 2004) created a conceptual model in which the competencies of the CNS role are described. The framework is called the three spheres of influence. The three spheres include the patient/client sphere, the nurses and nursing practice sphere, and the organization/system sphere. The framework provides flexibility and recognizes that CNS practice may be actualized differently based on the CNS specialty, setting, population, and/or organizational needs.

Components of the Job Description

In most health care agencies, components of a CNS or professional job description are organized by a preexisting format from the human resources department. A job description typically consists of several major components: a general overview or summary section, principal duties and responsibilities, qualifications, required and desired skills, and abilities/competencies (State Library of Ohio, n.d.). (See Appendix A.)

The Position Summary

The position summary is a brief description (three to five sentences) of the overall duties and responsibilities associated with the role. Position summaries may include information about the amount of freedom or independence the role has, existing partnerships, as well as to whom the person holding the job reports (State Library of Ohio, n.d.). The position summary helps answer the question, "Why does this job exist?"

Principal Duties and Responsibilities

The principal duties and responsibilities section is the heart of the job description. It captures *what you would do* or the fundamental purpose of the job and associated duties. Performance standards or competencies describe the expectations of how the job is to be performed (University of Pittsburgh, n.d.). Using an organizing framework—like the three spheres of influence—helps create distinction for the various functional role competencies and job responsibilities. The words used to describe the job role and actions should be higher-level verbs such as *compare* and *contrast, design, evaluate, establish, mentor,* and *lead.*

Required Qualifications

The required qualifications section should specify required educational preparation, experience, and licensure. The education qualification component can be challenging to write because of the different levels of educational preparation for CNSs that has occurred over the years. It wasn't until 1998 with the first publication of the *Statement on Clinical Nurse Specialist Practice and Education* that there existed a more definitive outline for classroom and clinical education specifically for the CNS (National Association of Clinical Nurse Specialists [NACNS], 1998). For recognition, many states now require CNSs to be certified by a professional nursing organization in addition to holding a graduate degree. Eligibility requirements for certification often include 500 supervised clinical hours completed within an educational program. Prior to the late 1990s, most programs' clinical hour requirement was less than 500 hours, leaving some long-practicing CNSs ineligible for selected certification examinations. In addition, many clinical specialty areas do not offer certification options at the advanced practice level. Addressing issues of certification in a job description requires some considered thought.

The goal of a job description is to ensure that each employee meets the minimum safe educational requirements to practice at an advanced level. Trying to achieve balance among educational preparation, legal requirements, and a sufficient number of available qualified candidates is tricky. The example job description demonstrates one method of achieving that balance in a state that does not have title protection (Appendix A). Minimum experience as a nurse and as a CNS needs to be spelled out. The title *CNS* denotes being an expert in a clinical specialty at an advanced level. Therefore, level of expertise in a clinical specialty and how that expertise will be achieved and maintained need to be described in the required qualifications section.

Skills and Abilities

The skills and abilities portion of the job description specifies minimum competencies required for job performance. Skills for the advanced practice nurse include leadership, communication, collaboration, mentoring, and leading change. These are the essential characteristics of the CNS role outlined in the NACNS *Statement on Clinical Nurse Specialist Practice and Education* (2004). Abilities are those personal characteristics an employee has that may be needed to excel in a job. A CNS should be able to demonstrate the ability to utilize evidence to develop, teach, guide, and implement practice standards and policies. These skills and abilities should be verified through a portfolio, recommendation letters, the interview process, and/or demonstration.

Desired Qualifications

The final components listed in the job description are those qualifications that are desired but not required. Desired additional qualifications can be used as a strategy to help determine the better candidate when two or more job applicants meet all the required qualifications for the job. Some examples of desired qualifications include certification in an area of clinical specialty, experience as a CNS greater than 5 years, and computer skills using various applications including word processing, presentation programs, and databases. Desired qualifications can often tip the scales during the hiring process if there is a competition between applicants with similar required qualifications.

Controversies and Practical Solutions

Educational preparation, key clinical experience, and reporting structure are essential components of any CNS job description; however, these content areas may create some controversy during the development phase. Defining educational preparation for a CNS can be challenging due to the historical and current variability of CNS educational programs across the country (Hamric, Spross, & Hanson, 2005). CNS educational programs today should be accredited and should address national recommendations for course content and clinical experiences outlined by the American Association of Colleges of Nursing *Essentials of Master's Education* (1996) and the NACNS *Statement on Clinical Nurse Specialist Practice and Education* (2004), including a minimum of 500 hours of supervised (by a CNS) clinical experience. The CNS applicant who has recently completed a graduate program that meets recommendations should be able to enter into CNS practice.

Performance evaluation may be used to determine any deficits that could be resolved through continuing education or continuing clinically precepted experiences. CNS applicants should possess a minimum level of nursing practice experience and expertise in the clinical specialty area. The expectation of demonstrated clinical expertise should occur within 6 months to 1 year of hire. Without this expectation, the CNS may have difficulty fully operationalizing the CNS role of expert clinical practitioner.

Another area of controversy includes reporting relationships. A CNS, as an advanced practice nurse, should report to a nursing administrator with an advanced degree. Variations on reporting relationships will exist, and reporting relationships are highly dependent on the organization's administrative structure. Within complex organizations, the primary need is for consistency in the reporting structure. By standardizing the reporting relationships, the CNS position is strengthened and supported throughout the organization.

Because the role of the CNS is essentially that of expert clinical practice and support for the bedside nurse in the provision of the highest quality nursing care, the CNS should lead clinical practice for the unit, program, or area. Partnering the CNS and the nurse manager provides optimal unit or program leadership. The CNS and the nurse manager work as partners to support the nursing clinical practice of the unit or across a program. Collaboration promotes best practices and supports positive nursing outcomes. Joint meetings to identify each partner's role, discuss potential concerns, and offer models of working CNS/nurse manager partnerships also help support the CNS and the nurse manager. Clearly articulating the CNS role components for nurse managers and other leaders may help decrease resistance to these partnerships. Illustrating the potential value and outcomes of successful partnerships will educate CNSs and nurse managers unfamiliar with each other's role and will help them work together successfully in the future.

Once consensus is reached regarding any controversial areas, the job description is complete. The next step is to submit the document to administration and human resources for final approval. While that review is under way, the group can begin to look at creating the interview process, orientation, and performance appraisal.

Using the CNS Job Description to Develop Other CNS Tools

A carefully crafted CNS job description that is based on national standards and reflects the needs for CNS practice in a particular organization becomes an invaluable foundation for the development of other tools related to the CNS role. The CNS core competencies and responsibilities in each of the three spheres of influence that are detailed in the job description provide a consistent structure for the CNS interview process, the CNS orientation program, and the CNS performance evaluation.

CNS Interview Process

Candidates for CNS positions should be initially screened to ensure that they meet the required qualifications for educational preparation and experience that are specified in the job description. Nursing directors can clarify whether a candidate has the appropriate master's degree by asking if the candidate had supervised clinical in a hospital/clinical facility and clinical experiences that incorporated components of the CNS role (i.e., a practice change project, transfer of evidence into practice). Those candidates who meet the required qualifications can be further evaluated though interviews, portfolio reviews, and letters of recommendation.

The interview process should have a broad base of participation from staff that will interface directly with the CNS, including the nursing director, nurse manager, staff nurses, other CNSs, and select multidisciplinary team members. Participation by multiple interviewers can be facilitated through the use of a structured interview tool with questions based on core competencies in each of the three spheres of influence. These questions will help evaluate the candidate's strengths in advanced practice skills of leadership, communication, collaboration, mentoring, and change management. For example:

Direct Patient Care

- Describe skills that are necessary to work with various groups.
- Talk about a time when you used these skills in a patient care situation. (team building/collaboration, communication, leadership)

Nursing/Nursing Practice

■ Give an example of a time when you used evidence or performance improvement to change nursing practice or standardize care at the institutional level. (leadership, clinical expertise, communication, problem solving, change management, mentor)

Organization/System

■ What issue do you think will have the most impact on the way nursing is practiced in the future? (professional development, leadership)

A structured recording tool should be used to allow interview participants to record their impressions of the candidates' answers. Portfolios can be very helpful in demonstrating the candidates' prior experiences and skill sets in many areas of CNS practice. Candidates can also be asked to provide brief educational presentations as a part of their interview with staff nurses.

CNS Orientation Program

The CNS orientation program is based on achieving competencies that are derived directly from the responsibilities listed in the CNS job description. The structural framework is again the three spheres of CNS practice. The orientation should also incorporate adult learning principles and be customized to meet the individual needs of the CNS orientee. At the heart of an orientation program is the guidance and mentoring of a CNS preceptor assigned to the orientee for the duration of the orientation period. Tools might include a CNS Skills Inventory and a Competencies/Resource List. The orientee could use the Skills Inventory to identify and prioritize areas for further development. The orientee and the CNS preceptor could use a Competencies/Resource List to identify aspects of the CNS role on which to focus during orientation and the corresponding resources that may be used to help the orientee achieve competency in those areas. The length of the orientation is customized according to the needs of the orientee. The orientee's achievement of the competencies is evaluated jointly by the orientee, the CNS preceptor, the nurse manager, and the nursing director. The orientee is also asked to evaluate the orientation program itself to facilitate program improvement. See Chapter 5 for more in-depth discussion of CNS orientation.

CNS Performance Evaluation

The annual evaluation of the performance of a CNS provides an opportunity to obtain feedback from the customer base. A useful tool could be a brief CNS Customer Survey that allows customers to rate the CNS's performance on some of the key role responsibilities and to rank the importance of each of those functions to the customer. CNSs may use a CNS Performance Evaluation Rating tool to self-assess their performance in all three spheres of influence: direct care, nurse/nursing practice, and organization/system leadership. The ratings are divided into four categories of performance: not met, approaching, solid performance, and exemplary. Sample behaviors are described under each category to assist in the rating process. The focus of behaviors in the three spheres will fluctuate for each CNS depending on the annual goals developed in partnership with the nursing director and the nurse manager partner.

The CNS job description is the starting point for the development of all of the tools described above. There are major advantages to this development approach. Since the job description is founded on national standards of CNS practice, the other tools are then aligned with the national standards. In addition, the consistent use of the same core competencies and role responsibilities in all of these documents sets a high standard for CNS performance while allowing for individual variation to meet the demands in different practice settings. Finally, the structural framework of the three spheres of influence defines and facilitates CNS participation in the full scope of CNS practice.

References

American Association of Colleges of Nursing. (1996). *The essentials of master's education for advanced practice nursing*. Washington, DC: Author.

Hamric, A. B., Spross, J. A., & Hanson, C. M. (2005). *Advanced practice nursing: An integrative approach* (3rd ed.). St. Louis: Elsevier Saunders.

National Association of Clinical Nurse Specialists (NACNS). (1998). *Statement on clinical nurse specialist practice and education* (1st ed.). Harrisburg, PA: Author.

National Association of Clinical Nurse Specialists (NACNS). (2004). *Statement on clinical nurse specialist practice and education* (2nd ed.). Harrisburg, PA: Author.

State Library of Ohio. (n.d.). *Job description components*. Retrieved September 9, 2007, from http://winslo.state.oh.us/publib/jobcomp.html

University of Pittsburgh-Office of Human Resources. (n.d.). *Components of the job description*. Retrieved September 5, 2007, from http://hr.pitt.edu/comp/jdcomponents.htm

CLINICAL NURSE SPECIALIST JOB DESCRIPTION:
POSITION SUMMARY/ESSENTIAL CHARACTERISTICS

The clinical nurse specialist (CNS) is the clinical leader for a program or area of nursing practice. The advanced knowledge and skills required for this role include clinical expertise in a focus area, evidence-based practice, collaboration, consultation, education, mentoring, and change leadership. These are essential to advance the practice of nursing and the professional development of nurses. The specialized knowledge and skills are used within three major areas of focus: patient/family, nurses and nursing practice, and the organization/system. The CNS and the nurse manager are partners in leading the nursing clinical practice area. The CNS coordinates and guides clinical activities/projects of nurses within a practice area. The CNS is accountable for collaborating with members of the health care team to design, implement, and measure safe, cost-effective, evidence-based care strategies. The CNS is responsible for maintaining current professional knowledge and competencies and contributing to the advancement of the practice of nursing at the unit/system, local, state and/or national and international level.

Responsibilities

Direct Patient Care

1. Serves as a reliable source of information on the latest evidence supporting cost-effective, safe nursing practices.
2. Collaborates with the multidisciplinary team using the nursing process to integrate the nursing perspective into a comprehensive plan of care for the patient/family.
3. Identifies and prioritizes nursing care needs for a select population of patients/families.
4. Conducts comprehensive, holistic wellness and illness assessments using established or innovative evidence-based techniques, tools, and methods.
5. Initiates and plans care conferences or programs for individual patients or populations of patients.
6. Designs and evaluates innovative educational programs for patients, families, and groups.
7. Identifies, collects, and analyzes data that serve as a basis for program design and outcome measurement.
8. Establishes methods to evaluate and document nursing interventions.

9. Evaluates the impact of nursing interventions on fiscal and human resources.

Nursing/Nursing Practice

1. Collaborates with others to resolve issues related to patient care, communication, policies, and resources.
2. Creates and revises nursing policies, protocols, and procedures using evidence-based information to achieve outcomes for indicators that are nurse-sensitive.
3. Identifies facilitators and addresses barriers that affect patient outcomes.
4. Leads clinical practice and quality improvement initiatives for a unit or a program.
5. Collaborates with nurses to develop practice environments that support shared decision making.
6. Assists the staff in developing critical thinking and clinical judgment.
7. Creates a nursing care environment that stimulates continuous self-learning, reflective practice, feeling of ownership, and demonstration of responsibility and accountability.
8. Collaborates with educational nurse specialists, educational nurse coordinators, and others on content and operational design of orientation, clinical competency, and other clinical educational program development.
9. Mentors nurses to acquire new skills, develop their careers, and effectively incorporate evidence into practice.
10. Provides input for staff evaluation.
11. Provides formal and informal education for nurses and other health professionals and health professional students.
12. Leads in the conduct and utilization of nursing research.

Organization/System Leadership

1. Consults with other units and health care professionals to improve care.
2. Leads/assists institutional groups to enhance the clinical practice of nurses and improve patient outcomes.
3. Develops, pilots, evaluates, and incorporates innovative models of practice across the continuum of care.
4. Designs and evaluates programs and initiatives that are congruent with the organization's strategic plans, regulatory agency requirements, and nursing standards.
5. Participates in need identification, selection, and evaluation of products and equipment.
6. Advances nursing practice through participation in professional organizations, publications, and presentations.

Required Qualifications

Education

Graduate degree (master's or doctorate) in nursing with a clinical focus. Graduate preparation must have included clinical application of the CNS role component.* If clinical application of the CNS role was not included in the candidate's master's preparation, a post-master's CNS certificate must be obtained within 3 years of date of hire to maintain employment in this classification.

Experience

■ Minimum 3 years clinical nursing experience required.
■ Clinical knowledge in specialty area. If hired in area with a substantially different clinical knowledge set, the candidate will be expected to demonstrate clinical expertise in the practice area within 6-months to a 1-year time frame.

Skills

■ Demonstrated skills at the level of an advanced practice nurse in leadership, communication, collaboration, mentoring, and change as evidenced by portfolio, recommendation letters, references, interview, and demonstration.
■ Demonstrated ability at the level of an advanced practice nurse to utilize evidence to develop, teach, guide, and implement practice standards and policies.

Desired Qualifications

Advanced Practice Certification as a CNS.
Certification in area of clinical specialty.
Clinical nursing experience within the last 5 years.
Computer skills using various applications: Internet, e-mail, word processing, presentation, and database.

*As defined by the National Association of Clinical Nurse Specialists. (2004). *Statement on clinical nurse specialist practice and education* (2nd ed.). Harrisburg, PA: Author. Curriculum recommendations on pp. 42–43.

3

Finding a Place in the Organization

Jan Powers

Clinical nurse specialists (CNSs) are vital to building a health care system that is evidence-based, patient-centered, safe, ethical, outcomes-focused, and cost-effective (Heitkemper, 2004). Sometimes, finding a place in the organizational structure can be a source of frustration for the new CNS. This is especially true with the changing nature of health care organizations. The following information will assist you in your quest for a CNS position that meets your own professional needs as well as the needs of an organization to provide safe, high quality, cost-effective care to patients.

Complexity of Health Care Systems

The complexity of health care systems has increased dramatically in the past several decades (McKeon, 2006). The intricate nature of health care requires multiple team members to manage patient care, making it imperative that effective communication and interprofessional collaboration occur. The culture within an organization will also determine its ability to function and produce high quality outcomes. A strong culture facilitates high performance. A system of shared values allows employees to apply these values to benefit the organization as a whole. The foundation of a strong culture in health care is trust among disciplines, collaboration, and communication (McDougall, 1987). Communication is that process of sharing information with people that increases their understanding. Trust and collaboration involve understanding and valuing each role's unique contributions and the ability to work together to attain the best outcomes for patient care (McDougall, 1987). Therefore, it is essential that all team members understand the responsibilities of all the roles so that they can effectively work together.

Different Disciplines and Roles

Different disciplines each have their own knowledge base, behaviors, and standards of practice (Orchard, 2005). Each member of the team brings a different set of values, personal experiences, and beliefs. In order to develop trust for collaborative practice to occur, role clarification and role valuing are required (McKeon, 2006).

A role is a set of behaviors that a person is expected to perform (McDougall, 1987). Roles need to be clearly delineated through job descriptions that provide the sets of expectations defining the roles. If roles are not clearly defined, role conflict may occur. Role conflict and role ambiguity create stress, diminish the effectiveness of the organization, and create extra work for the employee (McDougall, 1987). In a highly effective organization, all professionals are valued and recognized as possessing the intellectual and moral capital necessary to provide excellent patient care (McKeon, 2006).

The CNS is an integral part of an organization and brings a unique clinical focus to his/her practice. The CNS role historically involved many different roles, including leader, educator, researcher, and consultant. Because of these many different roles, the CNS role may be confused with other roles within an organization. It is imperative that a new CNS understand other roles in the organization and clearly delineate and explain to others the unique qualities of the CNS.

The CNS role may overlap with other roles such as educators, case managers, quality liaisons, clinical managers, and clinical pharmacists. The roles and goals of the CNS's practice must be clearly identified and defined for other disciplines to clearly understand. Therefore, it is imperative for the new CNS to not only articulate his/her roles and responsibilities, but to understand other roles within the institution and how to integrate his/her role into the institution. Variation of roles may exist among different institutions, so it is important to ascertain role functions and duties and be able to verbalize how the CNS can collaborate with each specific role.

Nursing Educator

The CNS role is often confused with the educator role; in fact, some institutions have attempted to combine the educator and CNS roles into one job category. This typically has not worked well and should be discouraged because the role of educator usually becomes the primary focus at the expense of the clinically expert role model aspects of the CNS role. A nursing educator role should be focused entirely on educating and training of nurses and nursing staff.

Case Manager

Case management is a collaborative process that assesses, plans, implements, coordinates, monitors, and evaluates options and services to meet an individual's health needs through communication and available resources to promote quality, cost-effective outcomes (Conger, 1996). Case managers may be referred to by different names or positions, such as care manager, outcomes manager, or care coordinator. This person guides patients through the complex health care process, providing responses to questions and connecting the patient and family to needed resources.

Quality Managers

Quality managers or liaisons use a comprehensive body of knowledge and are experts at quality agency regulations and data required to meet these mandated standards of practice. These experts in performance improvement and quality assurance should help guide and direct processes that promote safe, high quality, cost-effective patient care (Healthcare Quality, n.d.). The quality liaison also provides internal measurement of quality indicators and provides benchmarking for both internal and external quality indicators.

Nurse Practitioner

The nurse practitioner (NP) conducts physical examinations, orders and interprets laboratory results, selects plans of treatment, identifies medication requirements, and performs certain medical management activities for selected health conditions, usually with a focus on meeting primary health care needs (American Academy of Nurse Practitioners, n.d.).

These are just some examples of roles that may be present in any organization where a CNS may also be employed. Variations of roles exist within different organizations; therefore, it is important to ascertain role functions and duties and be able to articulate how the CNS is different from, yet can collaborate with, each specific role.

CNS Role Within an Organization

The essence of CNS practice is clinical expertise in a specialty area and expertise in nursing practice in the care of complex patients (National Association of Clinical Nurse Specialists [NACNS], 2004). CNS education includes content on role competencies within the spheres of influence (patient/client, nursing practice/nurses, system/organization). The CNS impacts patient outcomes directly through practice and indirectly through influence of practice at the bedside. The CNS assists staff in impacting practice by creating an environment that promotes the empowerment of nursing (DeBourgh, 2001). The CNS role models advanced nursing practice by interacting confidently with physicians, demonstrating flexibility in complex situations, incorporating feedback of others before reaching a decision, and demonstrating accountability (DeBourgh, 2001).

Through evidence-based nursing care standards and programs of care, a CNS influences nurses (NACNS, 2004). He/she can also influence systems to mobilize, change, or transform in order to facilitate expertly designed nursing interventions targeted toward achieving quality, cost-effective, patient-focused outcomes (NACNS, 2004). The application of the nursing process at an advanced practice level and execution of clinical decision making are integral to the role of the CNS. The CNS develops innovative solutions while acting as a change agent, assists nursing staff with decision making in clinical situations, and promotes evidence-based clinical practice and research to optimize clinical practice.

The CNS is a champion for evidence-based practice, clinical inquiry, and nursing research that aims to improve patient outcomes specifically related to nursing practice. The CNS disseminates current research-based literature and theories necessary for the advancement of patient care. The CNS also conducts cost-benefit analyses and promotes cost-effectiveness of interventions and process improvements along with product utilization to ensure desired outcomes and cost containment. The CNS contributes to the development of interdisciplinary standards of practice, guidelines of care, and system level policy. Utilizing evidence-based practice and resources, CNSs develop key tools and processes that support achievement of quality outcomes for specific populations and create innovative alternative solutions to system problems.

The CNS serves as a mentor and role model for the staff. The CNS must be proficient in interpersonal skills related to communication, collaboration, group process, conflict management, and negotiation.

Integration Into an Organization

Organizational behaviors help explain organizational socialization, group development, and role making (Krcmar, 1991). The CNS often enters into a job as the only CNS in the system. If there is more than one CNS in the system, it is typical that each CNS has a different area of specialization. When a CNS enters a system, he/she becomes a member of multiple groups within the system, including the nursing leadership team, specialty unit staff, CNS peer group, medical staff, and various multidisciplinary teams such as the coronary care team, oncology team, and rehabilitation team. Successful organizational entry depends on the new CNS making a smooth transition. This transition can be challenging as the new CNS needs to develop an understanding of the organization, including the culture, values, and history, as well as the personalities of dominant leaders (formal and informal) within the organization.

Some measured steps can be taken to ease the transition from newcomer to insider. To become an insider, a CNS must begin to recognize system norms and organizational behavior patterns, accept organizational reality, achieve role clarity, and locate oneself within the organizational context (Krcmar, 1991). Understanding organizational culture, values, and norms does not mean that a CNS must conform to the practices. It is easier to transition to an organization that holds the same values and beliefs; however, personal and organizational values do not need to totally coincide. Often a CNS may be hired to assist in changing the culture and values of an organization. If this is the case, the CNS must be an expert in the change process and be very strong in his/her values—this may not be an optimal climate for a new CNS.

Entry into a system is a process that may take considerable time and energy. The process must be planned and deliberate with a designated time frame (Krcmar, 1991). Issues regarding role establishment and role clarification begin to emerge as a CNS enters an organization. Therefore, it is important to understand organizational structure and roles. Lack of consistency in defining the roles and responsibilities of the CNS contribute to role ambiguity (Harrell & McCulloch, 1986), and a lack of role definition leads to broad interpretation of the CNS role (Krcmar, 1991). The new CNS will undoubtedly encounter differing role expectations, and others will place varying degrees of importance on those expectations (Krcmar, 1991).

Even while mastering the CNS role components, challenges often occur for a new CNS when entering into a position where other advanced roles or other disciplines may have overlapping areas of responsibility or areas of support. The new CNS may experience role conflict and therefore struggle between being what he/she wants to be and conforming to the views others hold of the role (Krcmar, 1991). A new CNS will need to determine expectations and be able to articulate the CNS role in order to provide and reinforce clarity. This is also true if the nurse has been in an organization in a different capacity before taking a CNS position—such as moving from staff nurse to CNS. In this situation, a new CNS must establish oneself in a different role within existing relationships, as others tend to view the CNS in his/her previous capacity. Reestablishing a new role in the organization will require multiple reminders and reinforcement by the new CNS.

Collaboration

Complex organizations require many different roles and multiple team members to effectively manage patient care. With multiple team members it is imperative that organizations require interprofessional collaboration. A new CNS must establish those collaborative relationships with nurses and other providers in order to establish goals and to implement a plan of care. Collaboration may be hampered by differences in professional perspectives that exist across health providers (McKeon, 2006). Successful collaboration includes mutual trust and respect, and understanding and support of each other's roles and responsibilities. Collaboration should involve a shared vision, a common goal, and problem-solving and communication skills. A trusting relationship is built upon mutual respect and understanding and the ability to be comfortable with blending territories and individual maturity (Kopser, 1994).

By using sound theoretical knowledge of the change process, a CNS has the ability to influence attitudes, modify behavior, and introduce new approaches to nursing practice (King, 1990). A CNS in collaborative practice fosters mutual support and networking through commitments to professional interdisciplinary organizations at the local, state, and national levels. Positive outcomes of collaborative practice affect patients and their families, nurses, physicians, hospitals, and all health care professionals, resulting in satisfaction, decreased time spent resolving complaints, and possible earlier detection of patient problems (King, 1990).

Collaboration among disciplines is extremely important. The most effective outcomes will be developed through a collaborative approach. A CNS needs to participate with the nurse manager to plan for and implement goals related to nursing practice. He/she should assist with identifying education needs and collaborating with nurse educators to develop targeted plans for education of nursing staff. Over time, the CNS will also develop mutually respected CNS–physician relationships.

A CNS also needs to help physicians understand the role. Physicians often relate better to the elements of an advanced practice role that is consistent with the medical model. The CNS role is often difficult for the physician to understand. CNSs emphasize autonomous nursing practice, and nursing is more than just following physicians' orders. While nurses value respect and mutual trust, physicians value clinical competence, willingness to help, and good communication (King, 1990). Physicians may feel uncomfortable with educated nurses; many physicians see all nurses as equal and don't recognize levels of practice expertise within nursing. Nurses and physicians work their entire professional career side by side without really understanding the other (King, 1990). A collegial relationship is built on shared knowledge, confidence, and mutual trust. In an egalitarian working situation, a well-functioning team uses individual strengths, talents, and values on behalf of the patient and family (King, 1990).

Sources of Stress

Overlapping roles and functions, role conflict, role ambiguity, staff turnover, and cost containment may blur professional boundaries (McDougall, 1987). Other sources of stress may involve a heavy workload, lack of participation in decision making, and territoriality problems.

Placement of a CNS in the organizational structure is an important consideration for a new CNS. The CNS does not have line authority (management authority), so one needs to earn the trust and respect of others to be effective. Since the CNS usually promotes change by virtue of expertise rather than authority, communication skills are critical. The CNS reporting structure should be outside of the unit or specialty area. If the CNS reports to a director or manager of a service area, this implies that the CNS "belongs to" that individual and may be used to meet the director's own agenda rather than being encouraged to meet the CNS's own clinical needs. Optimally the CNS should report to a chief nursing officer or a CNS manager who is also a CNS. This type of reporting structure will enable the new CNS to gain the mentoring needed and develop a collaborative partnership with the manager or director of the unit or area for which he or she is responsible.

All professionals need to be valued and recognized as possessing the intellectual and moral capital necessary to provide excellent patient care. Strife and tension arise in an environment where there is a lack of congruence in vision and mission or where organizational leaders are more profit-driven than patient-driven (Richmond, 2005). In these situations, professionals may compromise their own personal values.

Keys to Effective Integration

Advanced practice nurses can make a complex health care environment into a solution-oriented facility rather than a blame-focused facility (Richmond, 2005). It is imperative that a CNS be able to maintain tranquility when surrounded by chaos. A CNS can affect decision making by becoming a member of strategic committees. Effective participation in patient rounds is the most direct method of influencing patient care; it is important to use patient rounds to their maximum benefit.

Even while mastering CNS practice competencies, challenges often occur for the new CNS when entering into a position. The CNS may need to determine expectations and articulate the role of the CNS to provide role clarity.

For the CNS, changing roles within an organization or changing organizations can be a stressful time. However, this can and should be a very exciting and rewarding experience for everyone involved. There are many steps that the CNS can take to ease his/her integration into the new role and/or new system; these are presented in Table 3.1. Follow these key steps for a successful entry into an organizational structure.

Following these key steps when the CNS enters an institution will help ease the transition. These steps include meeting with nursing leadership, medical directors, educators, and other key individuals. These meetings are a forum to

---

3.1 Tips for Successful Integration of a New CNS Into a Health Care Organization

- Ensure that patient care and outcomes address quality and safety.
- Ensure that reporting structure allows independent, creative practice.
- Take time to build trusting relationships.
- Develop lines of communication with formal and informal leaders in the organization.
- Determine expectations of others and find ways to collaborate with other providers and staff.
- Value the norms and behavior patterns of the organization.
- Align with selected individuals within the organization to create peer groups.
- Be able to articulate the CNS role and practice competencies.
- Look for opportunities, such as at staff meetings, to explain the CNS role.

introduce yourself, explain your role, and lay the foundation for collaborative practice. A CNS should spend time working with units and groups related to the specialty in order to understand current practice and to build relationships. A CNS can also hold journal clubs, attend unit meetings, and offer fliers and brochures to help others understand the role of the CNS. A new CNS needs to take the time to establish relationships and build trust. This will lay the foundation for future initiatives.

Confidence in one's role is an important contributor to success. Gaining and sharing confidence is also enhanced by establishing relationships with professional colleagues outside the workplace—professional growth is essential. Being a lifelong learner and developing relationships with peers who share strategies that work in their own organizations allow a CNS a variety of avenues to expand his/her influence.

References

American Academy of Nurse Practitioners. (n.d.). *FAQ about nurse practitioners*. Retrieved August 25, 2007, from http://www.aanp.org

Conger, M. (1996). Integration of the clinical nurse specialist into the nurse case manager role. *Nursing Case Management, 1*(5), 230–234.

DeBourgh, G. (2001). Champions for evidence-based practice: A critical role for advanced practice nurses. *AACN Clinical Issues, 12*(4), 491–508.

Harrell, J. S., & McCulloch, S. D. (1986). The role of the clinical nurse specialist: Problems and solutions. *The Journal of Nursing Administration, 16*(10), 44–48.

Healthcare Quality Certification Board. (n.d.). *Certified Professional in Healthcare Quality (CPHQ) Program*. Retrieved August 25, 2007, from http://www.cphq.org

Heitkemper, M. (2004). Clinical nurse specialists, state of the profession and challenges ahead. *Clinical Nurse Specialist, 18*(3), 135–140.

King, M. (1990). Clinical nurse specialist collaboration with physicians. *Clinical Nurse Specialist, 4*(4), 172–177.

Kopser, K. H. (1994). Successful collaboration within an integrative practice model. *Clinical Nurse Specialist, 8*(6), 330–333.

Krcmar, C. (1991). Organizational entry: The case of the clinical nurse specialist. *Clinical Nurse Specialist, 5*(1), 38–42.

McDougall, G. (1987). The role of the clinical nurse specialist consultant in organizational development. *Clinical Nurse Specialist, 1*(3), 133–139.

McKeon, L. O. (2006). Safeguarding patients, complexity science, high reliability organizations, and implications for team training in healthcare. *Clinical Nurse Specialist, 20*(6), 298–304.

National Association of Clinical Nurse Specialists (NACNS). (2004). *Statement on clinical nurse specialist practice and education* (2nd ed.). Harrisburg, PA: Author.

Orchard, C. C. (2005). Creating a culture for interdisciplinary collaborative professional practice. *Medical Education Online, 10*(11), 1–13.

Richmond, T. (2005). Creating an advanced practice nurse-friendly culture. *AACN Clinical Issues, 16*(1), 58–66.

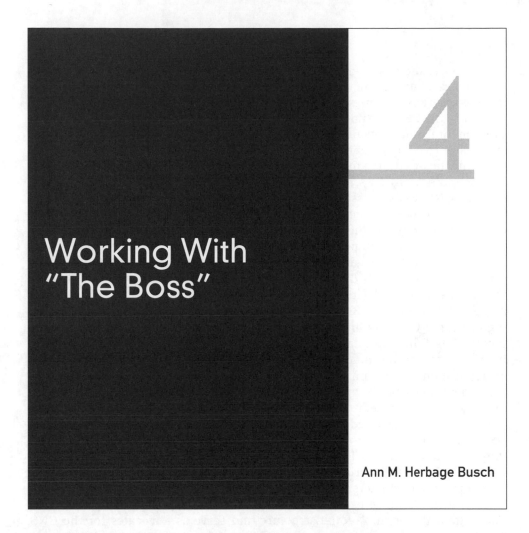

4

Working With "The Boss"

Ann M. Herbage Busch

Managing Up

The boss? What boss?! A motivated, independent, knowledgeable CNS might want to relegate dealing with a boss to a lower priority than dealing with the day-to-day patient issues. The patient does come first. However, in order to improve patient outcomes, dealing with the boss must also be high priority, especially for the novice CNS and the CNS in a new setting. What if the boss believes that the CNS should be added into RN staffing when staffing is short . . . and this happens 4 out of 5 days? Obviously, this CNS needs to deal with the boss or the CNS's goals will not get accomplished. The boss might have different ideas as to how to achieve improved patient outcomes, might prioritize differently, or might even have a different vision of the CNS job description and function than the CNS does. In addition, the boss has knowledge of economic pressures that will impact patient care and CNS role enactment. Therefore, dealing with the boss should be of utmost priority and has mutual benefits (Scott, 2007). Some management books call this "managing up" (Pearce, 2004). Managing your boss may initially sound a bit manipulative or Machiavellian; however, to be an effective employee and CNS, dealing with the boss is an important and legitimate reality.

Whether the boss is a nurse, a physician, a non-nurse and non-physician health care administrator, or an administrator without a health care background, there are certain activities and fundamentals the CNS should adopt in order to maximize the CNS role not only to survive but thrive. This chapter will cover the fundamentals that not only will help in dealing with the boss but will assist in successful role implementation and career achievement.

Many bosses draw a fine line between success and failure (Freedman, 2007). For example, at a CNS's annual performance review, instead of remembering that the CNS was successful in facilitating a dramatic decrease in surgical site infections, the boss remembers that the CNS did not develop a patient diabetic education booklet that the boss had as a priority. The boss then marks a satisfactory score for overall performance compared to the CNS's outstanding self-rating. To avoid this negative scenario, the CNS and the boss should initially discuss the CNS's goals during orientation. Hamric and Spross (1989) believe that the heart of the relationship between the CNS and the administrator may be goal setting together. By identifying problems and establishing and prioritizing goals, the CNS and the boss expose the common purpose that binds them together, and they can plan mutual activities to attain the goals. Goals should include items for the enhancement of the CNS's individual performance as well as department and organizational goals. Goal setting for 6 months with reasonable time frames may be more useful than for 12 months in the rapidly changing health care environment (Hamric & Spross, 1989). The goals should be written, measurable, and reviewed at least monthly with the boss to track progress, note accomplishments, and revise as necessary (Citrin & Smith, 2003). In addition, they should be shared with others in the organization who interface with the CNS to facilitate appropriate expectations of the CNS. This latter strategy may prevent future misunderstandings regarding the CNS role and priorities.

Misunderstandings can also be averted through supportive supervisors who understand the organizational structure and serve as advocates for the CNS. The boss can effectively introduce the CNS to the organization and key players (Hamric, Spross, & Hanson, 2005). Support from the boss is one of the strongest predictors of nurse job satisfaction (Scott, 2007). The boss is ideally someone who has credibility within the organization, is seen as a leader, works collaboratively with all departments, has influence over organizational resources, and has a different sphere of influence than the CNS (Hamric & Spross, 1989; Pearce, 2004). This administrator should also have expertise in management as well as nursing care issues and have a graduate level of education. If possible, having worked with CNSs previously and having a firm understanding of the CNS role and its value would add to the success of the administrator. It would also be a plus if the manager walked on water. Seriously, for a strong boss–CNS partnership, the individual would most likely have a nursing background with direct care and leadership experience. The boss could be a unit nurse manager or a vice president or director of nursing. However, if it is the former, potential conflicts could arise in that the CNS has the scope of the organization, not just the one unit, and must be allowed flexibility to accomplish goals that are outside the unit when appropriate. Conflicts may also arise if the boss is a busy vice president or director of nursing; this level of supervisor may be too busy with hospital administrative matters to give much supervision to the CNS. Finally, the boss might be a physician, a non-nurse and non-physician health care administrator, or an administrator without a health care background. If one of these situations is the case, it is imperative that the CNS be very clear about CNS and nursing roles so as not to become a "scut" worker, physician assistant, or jack of all trades. Although physicians have worked with nurses since medical school, there is often still a misunderstanding regarding the essence of nursing. By meeting regularly with the physician or other non-nurse boss to review role implementation, the CNS should be able to stay on track (Sparacino, Cooper, & Minarik, 1990). In addition, the CNS may want to perception check with CNS peers.

More Than One Boss

What if the CNS has more than one boss? There may be a "direct-line" boss and a "dotted line" to a boss with indirect responsibility. This often occurs when the primary boss is a non-nurse. In this instance, the CNS needs to be very aware of organizational politics and be very clear as to which boss has primary authority. Responsibility and accountability should be clearly delineated (Hamric & Spross, 1989). The primary boss has final approval of the CNS's goals, but input and approval should also be sought from the indirect boss.

Types of Supervision

The frequency of CNS and boss meetings and the amount of boss support the CNS requires vary with the qualities, experience, and education of the CNS. Most CNSs are committed professionals who are motivated to obtain personal success within the organization and who set difficult but achievable goals (Hamric & Spross, 1989). These qualities encourage supportive supervision, which gives the CNS freedom to determine many aspects of the role. However, supportive supervision does not mean that the CNS can do whatever she wants without regard to the organizational needs. With prospective communication and mutually agreed upon goals with the boss, this type of supervision allows a great deal of CNS autonomy in enacting the role with accompanying high CNS job satisfaction and still achieves organizational goals (Hamric & Spross, 1989). Despite there being a collegial and collaborative relationship between the CNS and the boss, the hierarchical chain of responsibility common to most health care organizations remains in place; the boss has administrative authority over job descriptions, operations, and evaluations (Hamric, Spross, & Hanson, 2005; Scott, 2007). For those CNSs with a lower level of maturity, less experience, or less commitment than the CNS described above, supervision can be increased to be more advisory and directive. This differential supervision takes the professional and role developmental level of the CNS into consideration. If this is the supervisory style used, the boss needs to be clear with the CNS soon after hire so that the CNS understands how to achieve greater autonomy in the future (Hamric & Spross, 1989).

How often should the supervisor have scheduled meetings with the CNS? New CNSs and CNSs new to organizations usually find it beneficial to meet with the boss for 1 hour weekly to clarify expectations, discuss progress, and seek guidance. Initially, the boss should be very specific and probe into the details of matters. Questions regarding strategies used, frustrations, areas of resistance, and organizational implications should be asked. Written goals, objectives, and explicit timelines should be reviewed in detail. Once the CNS demonstrates that problems are appropriately identified and prioritized, and goals, plans, intervention, and evaluation are expertly executed using excellent interpersonal skills and organizational finesse, the boss does not need to review future proposals in such detail (Hamric & Spross, 1989). In addition, frequency of meetings can be decreased. However, whether novice or experienced, all CNSs should still meet with their bosses periodically to receive ongoing feedback about clinical and leadership performance. Ongoing feedback makes explicit what the boss is thinking in terms of CNS performance and should encourage the CNS to make changes where needed. The CNS should also seek ongoing feedback from peers and should convey their valid information to the boss. Therefore, when the CNS's annual performance evaluation occurs, the CNS should not be hit with any surprises.

One significant point should be made regarding the CNS requesting meetings with the boss: Be cognizant of the boss's perception of these meetings. Sometimes the boss will see the increase in frequency of meetings as a sign that the CNS is weak and needy (Freedman, 2007). To avoid these perceptions, the CNS should have a legitimate reason to meet, make pertinent points concisely, omit whining, offer solutions, and conclude the meeting as quickly as possible.

Business Etiquette Fundamentals

Meetings with the boss can be stressful and even painful if a pleasant, healthy working relationship has not been established between the CNS and the boss. This relationship is one of the most important working relationships the CNS will have and deserves attention (Freedman, 2007). To establish an amiable relationship, "manage up" effectively, and be a great employee, the CNS should follow the nine fundamentals of business etiquette (Bruzzese, 2007; Citrin & Smith, 2003; Freedman, 2007; Pearce, 2004; Scott, 2007). See Table 4.1.

4.1   Business Fundamentals for the CNS

1. Know the organization and boss.
2. Make a first great impression and a lasting stellar reputation.
3. Be a good communicator.
4. Manage self.
5. Build good rapport with boss.
6. Understand and use attributes boss has to offer.
7. Offer CNS attributes to boss.
8. Treat boss fairly.
9. Give boss support, compliments, and appreciation.

First, the CNS needs to get to know the organization and boss (Pearce, 2004; Scott, 2007). Some topics to consider investigating: Is the organization for-profit or not-for-profit? Is it part of a larger multiorganizational structure? What are the patient demographics? What specialties are offered? What is the organizational culture? How does the CNS position fit into the organization? Are there other CNSs and a CNS peer group? Where does the boss fit into the organization? What are the boss's current goals, priorities, resources, and constraints? Is the boss laid back or hyperactive? Is afternoon the boss's most productive and approachable time of day? The CNS should try to better understand the boss in terms of role and personality. The CNS should observe, listen, and ask questions of other employees as well as take some time to talk with the boss about her background with the organization and her career goals. By learning more about the boss's world, the CNS gains insight into what the boss needs from the CNS and what might be expected. The CNS also gains insight into how to optimally interact with the boss. For instance, if mornings are not the best time of day for the boss, the CNS should not make an 8 a.m. appointment to discuss a controversial idea.

Second, the CNS needs to make a great first impression and then follow it up by building a lasting stellar reputation (Freedman, 2007). From the first interaction, impressions are made. The first impression might not even start with an in-person interaction but with an e-mail to a recruiter before the CNS is interviewed. Impressions often take into account dress, general grooming and appearance, language, body language, and more (Freedman, 2007). Seemingly inconsequential things such as a weak handshake can give a negative first impression. According to a 1971 study by Dr. Albert Mehrabian, a pioneer in the field of verbal and nonverbal communication, people are influenced less by what another says than how the person says it; 93% of a person's impact comes from things other than the actual words (Freedman, 2007). The CNS should be cognizant of the first impression she is making and ensure that it reinforces what she bills herself to be. After this initial impression is formed, a series of impressions are created over the next 6 months that coalesce into a reputation (Freedman, 2007). Once the reputation is formed, it is difficult to change, so the first 6 months of employment are especially critical. Creating a reputation can be seen as an opportunity for the new CNS. By consistently demonstrating the characteristics of integrity, dependability, trustworthiness, approachability, motivation, and being clinically expert, good at problem solving, and showing a positive attitude, the CNS will develop a reputation as a stellar integral member of the organization. Although building this reputation might sound somewhat formidable, it is built one day at a time. Once the reputation is formed, the CNS cannot slack off or become unapproachable, because over time, the reputation can change.

The third fundamental of being a great employee and managing up is to be a good communicator. Possibly foremost, this means being a good listener. Because the average rate of speaking is 125 to 150 words a minute, and listening comprehension is approximately 400 to 500 words a minute, there is a listening gap where the mind can wander (Bruzzese, 2007). Therefore, the CNS must make a conscious decision to listen intently and focus totally on the words and speaker. Making good eye contact with the speaker, smiling when appropriate, and summarizing what was just heard usually indicate a good listener (Bruzzese,

2007; Freedman, 2007). On the other hand, a poor listener often interrupts others. Interrupting implies that what the interrupter has to say is more important, and she is not truly listening (Bruzzese, 2007; Freedman, 2007). If the interruption is to finish the speaker's sentences, even if it is to give support to what he is saying, such as, "I know how you feel," it is considered rude and changes the focus from the speaker to the interrupter. Another indication of being a poor listener is fidgeting or doodling when someone else is talking. These activities indicate that the listener is not totally focused on the speaker and is distracted (Bruzzese, 2007).

Besides being a good listener, the good communicator does not ramble or dominate the conversation. Rambling may indicate nervousness, immaturity, insecurity, or a need to be the center of attention (Freedman, 2007), all attributes not associated with an effective CNS. A good communicator is aware that e-mails must be treated with respect: never put anything in writing that should not be seen by the boss or anyone else in the organization. Because each individual has a favored form of communicating, the CNS should discuss with the boss and then employ the style of communication the boss prefers. Is it e-mail, memos, sound bites, or face-to-face long discussions? If it is a written form of communication, the CNS must ensure that words are spelled correctly and proper grammar is used; if not, the CNS looks sloppy (Bruzzese, 2007; Freedman, 2007). By communicating effectively with the boss, the CNS facilitates a healthy working relationship and positively impacts her performance appraisal and career (Scott, 2007).

The fourth business fundamental for the CNS is to manage self and be the kind of employee bosses love (Freedman, 2007). This encompasses a myriad of elements from time to technology to attitude. One way the CNS manages self is by doing her job well. The CNS must perform the job that the boss wants the CNS to do, not necessarily what the CNS thinks she should do (Pearce, 2004); establishing goals together is the key to managing this potential dilemma. The CNS needs to meet all deadlines, keep her word, have good follow-through, and be a trusted and loyal ally. Time must be productively managed so that priorities are completed; there are only so many hours in a day, and the CNS often has more on the plate than is possible to accomplish. Also in managing self, the CNS needs to be prepared for all meetings, especially those with the boss. The CNS should arrive to meetings on time, have all necessary facts and details available, and present in an orderly objective fashion (Citrin & Smith, 2003; Pearce, 2004). Technology such as cell phones and e-mails needs to be managed; the CNS must establish rules with family and friends as to when to call or when messages can be returned. Personal e-mails should not be dealt with during business hours (Bruzzese, 2007). Finally, when managing self, an enthusiastic and positive attitude is one of the most important elements that bosses look for (Belker & Topchik, 2005; Citrin & Smith, 2003; Freedman, 2007). The CNS with a positive attitude demonstrates it by starting work on time, working hard and showing that she cares about the job, not getting defensive when constructive criticism is offered, not gossiping, using a sense of humor, and not blaming others when things do not work out as expected (Bruzzese, 2007; Freedman, 2007). The bottom line for fulfilling the fourth fundamental business skill is that the CNS manages self so well that the boss's job is easier: multiple demands are not made on the boss's time to manage the CNS.

Fundamental business skill number five entails having the CNS build a good rapport with the boss. Since the relationship with the boss is one of the most essential components to nursing job satisfaction, this fundamental deserves attention and time to develop. Having regularly scheduled meetings with the boss provides time and a forum to better understand each other, establish a bond, and thereby work more effectively together. Scott (2007) suggests viewing the boss as a client or patient since nurses extend themselves to meet their patients' or clients' needs and should be doing the same for the boss. Showing respect for the boss will encourage the boss to respect the CNS (Pearce, 2004). Sometimes people do not bond right away. If this is the case with the CNS and the boss, the CNS should persist in trying to develop rapport and remember that developing strong relationships with friends and family takes months and sometimes years (Freedman, 2007).

The sixth business fundamental for the CNS is to understand and use what the boss has to offer (Pearce, 2004). The boss will have attributes and organizational power that the CNS will not have. For instance, the boss might have easier access to power and influence, more experience, greater status, more control over resources, a broader vision of the organization, and greater knowledge of the politics and inner workings of the organization. When working on developing and achieving goals, the CNS should tap into these areas as appropriate. For instance, the boss should be accountable for facilitating a proper orientation and successful integration into the organization, arranging for an office and other essential items such as a beeper and a computer, providing another viewpoint on issues, providing guidance in dealing with a difficult situation, and providing active support on projects. The boss should also be expected to provide clear expectations of the CNS role, give ongoing feedback regarding the CNS's performance, and complete the CNS's annual performance appraisal.

Just as the boss has attributes to offer the CNS, the CNS has attributes to offer the boss (Pearce, 2004). This is business fundamental number seven. Some CNS attributes include clinical expertise, a greater and more detailed understanding of the day-to-day issues relating to the team and patients, more up to date knowledge regarding clinical issues, and a more informal relationship with nurses and other health care team members. The CNS should keep the boss informed of developments in her work so that the boss does not hear of them from others; the boss wants to hear it from the source and not be surprised. In addition, by keeping the boss informed, the CNS demonstrates a strong sense of responsibility and the ability to communicate clearly. The CNS should also offer to be the link to interpret economic realities and administrative decisions to staff nurses and clinical realities to administrators (Hamric & Spross, 1989). Anything the CNS can do to make the boss's job easier will be valued by the boss (Freedman, 2007). By offering to contribute and work hard for the team as well as by acknowledging appreciation for any opportunity to learn from the boss, the CNS sets this business fundamental into action.

The eighth business fundamental for the CNS is to treat the boss fairly: never criticize or complain about the boss and never go over the boss's head (Pearce, 2004). Despite choosing a "safe" person in whom to vent frustrations or complaints about the boss, this information seems to eventually get back to the boss. The boss then loses trust in the CNS, which undermines the whole working relationship. If the CNS has an issue with the boss, the issue should be openly discussed with the boss in a scheduled meeting and suggestions for resolution given. While criticism of the boss can break the working relationship, so can going over the boss's head. In the business world, the hierarchical chain of command should be respected and protocol should be followed when communicating; otherwise the CNS alienates herself not only from the boss but also from the boss's colleagues (Pearce, 2004). The CNS should go over the boss's head only in very serious circumstances, for instance, with harassment. If this type of situation occurs, the CNS should first seek guidance from the human resources department.

The ninth and final business fundamental in dealing with the boss is that the boss needs support, compliments, and appreciation just as the CNS does (Bruzzese, 2007; Pearce, 2004). Support can be given in ways such as assisting the boss with her priority project, telling others about the boss's strengths, and functioning as an exemplary CNS in the organization. Compliments should be sincere, specific, and not manipulative. Legitimate appreciation can put a smile on the boss and brighten everyone's day.

Following these nine business fundamentals may not be enough to guide the CNS to successful dealings with the boss if the boss has a personality that is truly toxic (Lubit, 2004). If the boss is more than difficult, the CNS can fall into common but unhelpful coping methods such as avoiding interaction, calling in sick, or quitting the job (Scott, 2007). Instead of coping in these ways, the CNS should read Lubit's book (2004) or one of the many other books on dealing with difficult bosses and implement suggested strategies. If this approach does not help the situation, the CNS is advised to seek advice from a professional in the human resource department (Scott, 2007).

Conclusion

Dealing with the boss may initially seem to take time away from dealing with important patient issues. However, dealing with the boss is a crucial and legitimate concern, which will actually facilitate and provide more time for improving patient outcomes in the long run. By "managing up" effectively, the CNS can maximize CNS role implementation. In addition, the CNS and the boss can develop a successful, strong, and mutually beneficial relationship.

References

Belker, L. B., & Topchik, G. S. (2005). *The first-time manager* (5th ed.). New York: American Management Association.

Bruzzese, A. (2007). *Forty-five things you do that drive your boss crazy . . . and how to avoid them.* New York: Penguin Group.

Citrin, J. M., & Smith, R. A. (2003). *The 5 patterns of extraordinary careers: A guide for achieving success and satisfaction.* New York: Crown Business.

Freedman, E. (2007). *Work 101: Learning the ropes of the workplace without hanging yourself.* New York: Bantam Dell.

Hamric, A. B., & Spross, J. A. (1989). *The clinical nurse specialist in theory and practice* (2nd ed.). Philadelphia: W. B. Saunders.

Hamric, A. B., Spross, J. A., & Hanson, C. M. (2005). *Advanced practice nursing: An integrative approach* (3rd ed.). St. Louis, MO: Elsevier Saunders.

Lubit, R. H. (2004). *Coping with toxic managers, subordinates . . . and other difficult people.* Englewood Cliffs, NJ: Financial Times Prentice Hall.

Pearce, C. (2004). How to . . . manage your boss. *Nursing Times, 100*(12), 72–73.

Scott, D. E. (2007). Collaboration with your boss: Strategic skills for professional nurses. *South Carolina Nurse, 14*(1), 21.

Sparacino, P.S.A., Cooper, D. M., & Minarik, P. A. (1990). *The clinical nurse specialist: Implementation and impact.* Norwalk, CT: Appleton & Lange.

Moving
Forward

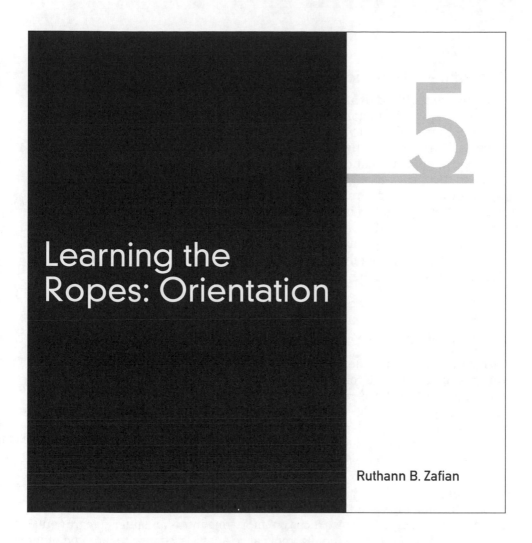

Learning the
Ropes: Orientation

Ruthann B. Zafian

Be Proactive: Ask for What You Want During Your Orientation and Beyond

You create your opportunities by asking for them.

—Patty Hansen, 2005

How exciting! You're about to accept your first job as a clinical nurse specialist (CNS)! Start creating your opportunities for success the moment you accept the job. Now is the time to start negotiating your orientation so you meet the people you need to know and start analyzing the corporate culture of your new work environment. It doesn't matter if you're a novice or an experienced CNS. It doesn't matter if you're new to the institution or have worked there for years. You know your strengths and weaknesses. You know what it is that you bring to the table. You know your learning needs and learning style. So be proactive right from the start and ask for what you need in your orientation. This is the time when your schedule will be the most flexible, before you get caught up in assignments, meetings, and clinical consultations. So take full advantage of it and learn everything you can.

The Value of Generic Orientation Classes

You may be required to attend hospital-wide, generic, or Nursing Department orientation programs, along with a variety of other hospital workers including the staff nurses. Though you may feel some of these classes are very basic, unnecessary, and not directly applicable to your work, don't fight it. There will be some pearls of information taught that you will find useful in some manner. Some of these classes are required by state or federal agencies, and all of them will afford you the opportunity to experience the orientation programs that are provided for new staff nurses. You need to know what they are being taught if you hope to exert influence in the nursing/nursing practice sphere (National Association of Clinical Nurse Specialists [NACNS], 2004). This is also an opportunity to start analyzing the quality of information provided to new nurses and the relationships that the Nursing Department has with other departments.

So, What Is It That You Do? What's a CNS?

"What does a CNS do?" Be prepared, because you're going to be asked to answer this question—or some form of it—over and over again. This may be your first opportunity to establish relationships with colleagues in the organization/systems sphere (NACNS, 2004) of your hospital. These first-impression meetings are very important. You'll need to have your 3-minute hip-pocket speech ready. You may even want to write it out so you can really hone your message, though your answer may differ based on who is asking the question. If a physician or an administrator were to ask the question, I'd say something like: "My focus is on optimizing clinical quality, patient/staff safety, and patient/family outcomes. I do this by helping nurses and other health care providers to understand and use evidence-based practice. I also focus on improving intra- and inter-departmental systems using appreciative inquiry, root cause analysis, change theory, and other quality improvement techniques."

If a staff nurse asked me the question, I'd say: "I'm here to make it as easy as possible for you to provide excellent patient care. I'll do this by making sure you have the information and knowledge you need to provide care. If you need to learn a new procedure, I can help. If you need information about a patient's diagnosis that you haven't seen before, I can help. I'll also be your advocate. I believe your voice needs to be heard when new equipment or processes are being evaluated. But first I need to know what you think about your work here, what works well, and what needs improvement. I need you to teach me, so I can help you."

What would you say? Whatever your message, make sure you have it on the tip of your tongue when asked, because you will be asked the question over and over. When I took on my first job as a CNS, I had a scheduled appointment to meet the Chief of Cardiac Surgery. As I anticipated, he asked me the "What's a CNS?" question. I explained my role. He looked perplexed for a moment and then he asked, "So, do I now have to go to you when I'm having trouble finding a bed for my patient?" I paused, pretended to wipe sweat from my brow, and said, "Thankfully no. That's not my role." Be prepared for questions like these by anticipating the interests and issues that are important to the person you'll be meeting with. Though I was not the person in charge of bed assign-ments, I quickly assured the chief of service that I would help optimize nursing care, system efficiencies, and patient outcomes so that the patients would move from ICU to telemetry to discharge in a timely and efficient manner. Essentially, I would help optimize patient throughput so beds would be available for the next surgical case. He nodded and seemed satisfied with that answer.

You also need to get used to saying, "I don't know, but I'll find out and get back to you." As a novice in the CNS role and perhaps a novice to the institu-tion, you may find yourself in the uncomfortable position of being asked one or several questions during these encounters, the answers to which you'll have no idea. But that's okay. No one expects you to have all the answers. They will, however, expect that you will follow through and be 100% reliable. So if you say, "I'll get back to you," make sure to keep your promise. You may also get stumped by some of the questions you'll be asked. When I was orienting to my first job as a CNS, I met with the Chief of Trauma Services. He asked me, "What's your philosophy of Nursing?" I never expected that question from a doctor and it re-ally took me by surprise. I'm sure I gave him the "deer in the headlights" look for at least 5 seconds, but then I regained my composure. I remember mumbling something about incorporating aspects of several nursing models into my ap-proach to clinical practice. Today, I would be much better prepared to speak about the American Association of Critical-Care Nurses (AACN, 2005) synergy model for patient care driving my philosophy of patient care and the principles of Pat Benner's (2001) *Novice to Expert* research as my guide to assessing the skills of staff nurses.

Try to end each one of these introductory meetings with two questions: (a) "If I have a question about something that involves your department, who would you like me to call?" Always try to leave with a phone number and contact person's name; and (b) "Now that you know a bit about my role, can you think of projects already in progress or coming up in the future where I could be of help?"

Find Yourself a Mentor

Make sure to spend a few hours shadowing other CNSs who work in your hos-pital. It's important to see how they enact the role and important to establish these relationships with your peers. Many times, these CNSs will be your great-est allies and sources of information about the inner workings and politics of the institution. When you meet with the other CNSs, ask how they quantify and qualify their work. If the CNSs in your hospital meet regularly to share infor-mation and support one another's work, make sure you attend these meetings.

Because even the most pro-CNS institutions employ a limited number of CNSs, and sometimes only one per specialty, it's easy to feel isolated. Make con-tact and stay in touch with your peers. Seek out one or more of these CNSs as your mentor. If you are the only CNS at your institution, consider someone in nursing education or administration as your mentor. The person you choose as your mentor should be someone who is open to a mentoring relationship with you, someone with whom you can communicate easily, and someone who has leadership or operational qualities that you admire. Even if that CNS works in a completely different specialty area of nursing, the CNS can help you acclimate to your new role. Time management may be a topic you might want to discuss with your mentor. Unlike the role of a staff nurse, the CNS job is never ending. You don't get to hand off your responsibilities to the next shift nurse at the end of your day. You will have multiple responsibilities, a variety of people competing for your time, and priorities that need rearranging daily (and some days, hourly). Most CNSs are exempt or salaried employees, and it will be easy to find yourself doing many more hours than you should. Be mindful of what's important, what's imperative, and what can wait. Though there may be days where you stay after normal business hours and do extra, be sure to take that time back. Don't allow yourself to get sucked into the job too much. Make sure to maintain your work-life balance.

Also, try to find out if there is a regional CNS group that meets regularly in your area. This is especially important if you are the only CNS at your institution. You need the support of someone who understands the unique and challenging role of the CNS. It's very interesting to speak with CNSs from other institutions and compare and contrast the implementation of their roles. It's gratifying to know how many projects and issues you have in common.

Get to Know Your Customers

Build in plenty of time to spend shadowing some of the staff nurses you'll be working with on all shifts. You need time to make sure you get to know them and their needs. They in turn need time to get comfortable with you. Though CNS job descriptions vary from institution to institution, almost all call for spending a considerable amount of time working within the patient/client and nursing/nursing practice spheres of influence (NACNS, 2004). So working with staff during your orientation will be very valuable to your future success. As you spend time observing and getting to know the staff nurses with whom you'll be working, simply offer your help. Ask how you can help with patient care in the short term (France, 2006). Use humor and remain nonconfrontational, even when challenged with skeptical or rude remarks. When I started at my current job, I asked one ICU nurse how I could help her. She smirked and replied: "So are you ready to get your hands dirty?" I winked and responded: "Sure, at least to get my gloves dirty." The nurse may only allow you to assist with something simple like patient positioning at first, but as the nurse sees you day in and day out, the staff nurse will become more comfortable with you and eventually trust you enough to ask for real help or information.

"Seek First to Understand, Then to Be Understood"

You may be very eager to get in and prove yourself, make a difference, and show people what you know. But when you are new to the CNS role, I suggest you tread very lightly at first. These first encounters with the staff nurses are your one and only chance for first impressions. Your demeanor needs to be friendly and that of a learner. Keep this motto from Stephen Covey (2004) in mind: "Seek first to understand, then to be understood." In reality, you will learn as much from the staff nurses as they will learn from you. If nurses are to eventually learn from you, they will first need to feel emotionally safe around you. If you are speaking with a nurse or other colleague and you start to sense that the person does not feel safe, it is in your best interest to change tactics to help the other feel safe again (Patterson, Grenny, McMillan, & Switzler, 2002). You need to understand and show respect for strengths and frustrations. You may see behaviors and styles of practice that you feel need to be changed, but while you are so new to the CNS role, avoid being critical until you understand these important customers better. Of course, if you see unsafe practice, you'll need to step in, but your approach in these situations is key to future success. Understand that some folks will be intimidated by you or will resent you before they even meet you. This is not unusual in some staff nurses and even some nurse managers who do not have the degree(s), experience, or credentials that you have. Again, tread lightly and help these colleagues to feel safe around you. Show appreciation for the knowledge and experience that these nurses bring to the table, and those barriers to collaboration will disappear eventually.

If you're in a situation where you are transitioning from the role of staff nurse to CNS in the same organization or within the same unit or service, be assertive and set limits as you transition to your new role. You may be tempted to do many of the things you did as a staff nurse because that is your comfort zone. Others may have difficulty understanding your non-clinical responsibilities and even expect that you will supplement staffing numbers. In time you will find a new comfort zone in the role of the CNS. Do not allow staff or managers to think of you as a per diem staff member. You certainly want staff nurses to request clinical consultations with you and ask for your help at the bedside, but it is not your job to replace the nurse at the bedside. I have heard of programs that require CNSs to provide direct care and take a staff assignment for a predetermined set of days or hours each month. The rationale is to ensure you are able to maintain your clinical proficiency. Though I do not believe this is the best use of the CNS, if you agree to this when you are hired into the role, go with it, but resist being used as a supplemental staff member on other days. You have other important work to do beyond direct patient care. That work requires a flexible schedule for meetings, literature reviews, issue investigation, and consultations with members of the multidisciplinary health care team.

Avoid Role Ambiguity

Request weekly meetings with your director/supervisor for at least the first month or two, then continue to meet at least monthly during your tenure. This is essential to stay focused and in order to avoid role ambiguity. Role ambiguity arises when the post holder and/or other stakeholders are unclear about their conception of the role or hold different conceptions of it (Jones, 2005). The role of the CNS overlaps somewhat and also complements the roles of many other health care team members: the manager, the educator, and the nurse practitioner. If the CNS is unclear about his/her role within the organization, then the CNS will not be able to present him/herself confidently and will falter during this critical transition time. Your director or supervisor is the person with whom you need to negotiate the expectations of your role. You will also need the support of your director or supervisor to reinforce that description and differentiation of your role to others on the team. When I began my current role as cardiovascular CNS, I remember one of our nurse educators asked me to explain the difference between the roles of the CNS and the nurse educator. We had a nice discussion about the differences and the areas where our roles might overlap. She and I have always worked well together and have had no difficulties with role clarity. However, I remember speaking to my director about that discussion between the nurse educator and myself and was surprised at the alarm that sounded in her voice as she recounted the role ambiguity problems that had plagued the person who was in the cardiovascular CNS role before me. My director was determined not to allow that to become a problem again and set about making sure I, along with others on the team, knew what her role expectations were (for all of us).

As stated above, you may be expected to spend a certain number of hours each week or month providing direct patient care to maintain your clinical skills. Others may expect you to keep a record of your time and activities to ensure you are allocating enough of your time to being available to the staff. Make sure you discuss these role expectations with your director early in your orientation. If possible, use technology to your advantage. Set up databases or word documents to track your projects and goals. In my current position, I was able to have the Information Systems department build a feature into our computer order-entry system where anyone on staff can order a CNS consult with me regarding a specific patient. It just takes a few clicks of the computer mouse. This gives the nursing staff an easy way to initiate consults with me. Since I cover several different inpatient units, I also find it very helpful at the end of the year to run reports from this system that spell out the number of consults I get from each unit, the reason for the consult, and who initiated the consult. Explore other ways that the technology available in your institution might be helpful to you. For instance, does your hospital have an electronic incident reporting system? Whether the system for these reports is paper or electronic, is it possible for you to have access to the reports? It will help you identify learning needs and issues that need further investigation. You may need to negotiate access to this information via your director. If you have e-mail and internet access in your office, be sure to sign up to automatically receive e-newsletters from organizations associated with your work, such as your state hospital association or specific nursing organizations. I subscribe to several e-newsletters and I read them regularly. Keeping current on issues and research in your specialty is essential.

Access to information is crucial to your success as a CNS. Your director needs to understand that you need to be kept informed about a wide variety of issues affecting your areas. This includes information specific to the role and functions of managers. You may not be involved in the decisions surrounding these issues, but it is essential that you are aware of issues that may stress the staff or the patients you work with. You may need to present a persuasive argument to achieve this. Your director needs to know the benefits of keeping you in the loop. It is important that he or she trust in your discretion regarding sensitive topics and also that you understand the boundaries of your input and influence. If you are unsure whether the information being shared with you is strictly confidential or ready for wider distribution, be sure to ask. Also, don't be afraid to ask to be included on projects or committees that are of interest to you. There will be times when you learn about a new initiative that you find objectionable. You may want to ask if the topic is negotiable before sharing your objections to the plan with your director. For example, at my particular worksite we had avoided hiring graduate nurses (GNs) into the critical care areas for several years, but because of staffing shortages, management recently felt it was necessary to allow GNs this option. When I was informed about this, my first question to the director was, "Is this a done deal or are you asking for my opinion about the plan?" I was told this was a done deal, so in spite of my significant reservations about the plan, my response was to advise the director about what would be needed to successfully support the new ICU GNs to achieve competency, staff satisfaction, retention, and to maintain patient safety.

As you and your director come to a consensus about your role, begin to develop SMART goals. You should be able to start formulating these goals about a month or two after you've started and have begun to understand the priorities within your service line. SMART is an acronym for: (S) Specific, (M) Measurable, (A) Attainable, (R) Realistic, and (T) Tangible or Timely (Donahue, 2007). An example of a poorly worded goal is: "I will improve the quality of hand-off reports within my service line." A better goal might be: "By the end of this month, I will complete a survey of both groups of staff members (anesthesia and the post-cardiac surgery ICU, for example) regarding the issues surrounding hand-off report quality and develop a plan of action."

There is one other topic you may want to discuss with your director. If there was a CNS in your position previously, it is important for you to understand his or her legacy. Was that person well liked and successful, or was that person unsuccessful in the role and why? You may encounter more opposition from staff members if that last CNS was unable to win the respect of the staff or leadership team. If the previous CNS was well liked, I would ask staff members what it was that made that CNS successful. Liked or disliked, the ghosts of CNSs past may haunt you, but you will be more prepared to deal with this legacy if you understand the impressions that were left behind.

Build a Strong and Diverse Network of Professional Contacts

You'll need to determine who your primary and secondary customers are. Some will be obvious, like those within your own service line: your director, the nurse manager(s), the nurse educator(s), physicians, advanced practice nurses, physician assistants, and the staff nurses (who may be your toughest critics). Others may not be so obvious: the manager of the respiratory therapists, the manager of medical records, and so forth. Remember you are entering a role where you will need to negotiate within all three CNS spheres of influence (NACNS, 2004). Your work in the organizational/systems sphere will require your ability to influence decisions well beyond your service line. It's important that you spend time learning about the needs of all of these customers. Learn what your primary customers' needs or wants are, and make those your first projects. Some will have absolutely no idea what to do with you, and others will have extensive ideas.

Your relationship with the nurse manager(s) with whom you'll be working most closely can make or break you. Any change process you want to move forward that involves staff nurses will be in jeopardy unless you have the visible support of the nurse/unit manager, the person with line authority. CNS job descriptions vary greatly from person to person and from institution to institution, but one variable remains fairly constant. Every CNS is a change agent, and many CNSs work without direct authority. So your professional network and alliances will be vital to your ability to move agendas forward. I find face-to-face meetings much more productive than phone conversations, especially when the subject matter might be controversial. I use e-mail for updates and FYIs and for setting up meetings, but if topics need to be discussed and decisions made, I prefer meeting directly with the person or persons involved.

Once you've met most of your primary customers, arrange introductory meetings with folks outside your immediate service line and outside the Department of Nursing, for example, Respiratory Therapy, Pharmacy, Purchasing, Library, Quality Management, Physician Chiefs of Service, Medical Records, IT Services, ED, and so forth. Again, these folks may be very helpful as you start working on house-wide projects or teams. When you attend meetings, if there is anyone in the room that you haven't met before, walk right up and introduce yourself. Build yourself a reputation for being friendly, assertive, and confident (Sullivan, 2004).

Reserve Time for Reflection

It's tough being a novice again, but anytime you take on a new role or a new job you'll return to being a novice for a while. The good news is that because you have some experience behind you and the benefit of your master's program, you'll probably advance out of the novice stage fairly quickly. Still, you may not feel completely comfortable with your new role for a full year. This is a new and expanded role for you. The politics of the CNS role can be very challenging and the stress can wear you down. It's important to take time every day to decompress, reflect, and renew. How? That's for you to decide. Whether it's a walk outside at lunchtime or a few minutes in your office with your favorite music playing, make sure you find some time for you.

It may be helpful to keep in contact with some of your graduate school professors or those who graduated from the CNS program with you. Support each other and share your experiences. They may be dealing with or have dealt with similar challenging situations and have some pearls of wisdom for you. The benefits of building a large, strong foundation of professional contacts should not be underestimated.

Relationships

I can't overemphasize that the strength of your relationships with your director and your customers is your greatest asset. Develop an ever-present "I'm here to help" attitude and check your ego at the door. It may take a while before you're given responsibility for projects or committee work. Be patient and prove your ability with whatever projects come your way. The projects you are most interested in will come in time if you do well with the assignments that are handed to you. It's all about putting the patients and families first and mentoring other health care professionals and workers to do the same. Just as with any job, there will be days when you leave work feeling like you've really made a positive impact and other days where you leave feeling frustrated and dejected. Find constructive outlets for your own frustrations at the job and always try to maintain a cool head and a professional demeanor. Raising your voice, complaining, or blaming others may get you attention, but it will not get you closer to where you need to go today or in the future. For some great advice in handling difficult situations and conversations, I suggest reading the book *Crucial Conversations: Tools for Talking When Stakes Are High* (Patterson et al., 2002).

Summary

1. Be proactive: Ask for what you want during your orientation.
2. Attend the generic orientation program and learn everything you can from it.
3. Be articulate regarding the CNS role and what you bring to the table.
4. Find a mentor: Shadow other CNSs.
5. Get to know your primary customers and help them feel safe around you.
6. "Seek first to understand, then to be understood" (Covey, 2004).
7. Avoid role ambiguity and be SMART goal oriented.
8. Build a strong and diverse network of professional contacts.
9. Take time every day to decompress, reflect, and renew.
10. Nurture strong relationships with your peers and customers.

References

American Association of Critical-Care Nurses. (2005). *AACN synergy model for patient care*. Retrieved June 6, 2007, from http://www.aacn.org/WD/Certifications/content/SynModel. pcms?menu=Certifications

Benner, P. (2001). *From novice to expert: Excellence and power in clinical nursing practice*. Menlo Park, CA: Addison-Wesley.

Covey, S. (2004). *7 habits of highly successful people: 15th anniversary edition*. New York: Simon & Schuster.

Donahue, G. (2007). *Top achievement: Creating S.M.A.R.T goals*. Retrieved June 22, 2007, from http://www.topachievement.com/smart

France, N.E.M. (2006). Socializing clinical nurse specialist students for practice. *Clinical Nurse Specialist, 20*(4), 97–99.

Hansen, P. (2005, November). *In Prevention, pNA*. Retrieved July 30, 2007, from InfoTrac OneFile via Thomson Gale: http://find.galegroup.com/ips/infomark.do?&contentSet= IAC Documents&type=retrieve&tabID=T003&prodId=IPS&docId=A142476634&source= gale&uerGroupName=n0008&version=1.0

Jones, M. L. (2005). Role development and effective practice in specialist and advanced practice roles in acute hospital setting: Systematic review and meta-synthesis. *Journal of Advanced Nursing, 49*(2), 191–209.

National Association of Clinical Nurse Specialists (NACNS). (2004). *Statement on clinical nurse specialist practice and education* (2nd ed.). Harrisburg, PA: Author.

Patterson, K., Grenny, J., McMillan, R., & Switzler, A. (2002). *Crucial conversations: Tools for talking when stakes are high*. New York: McGraw Hill.

Sullivan, E. J. (2004). *Becoming influential: A guide for nurses*. Upper Saddle River, NJ: Pearson Education.

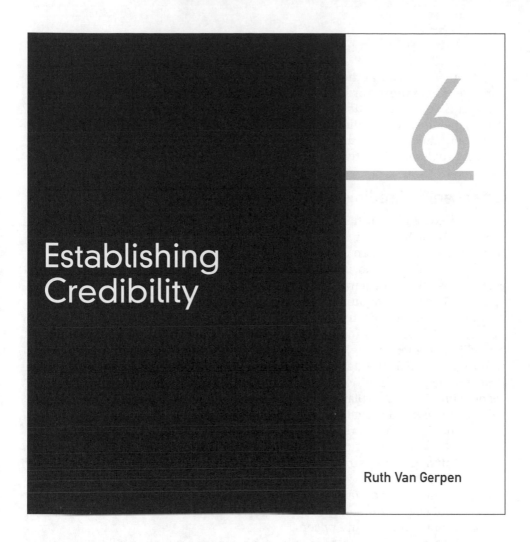

6

Establishing Credibility

Ruth Van Gerpen

Gloria has recently completed her master's in nursing program as a clinical nurse specialist (CNS) and has accepted a CNS position at a medical center in her community. Prior to graduation, Gloria worked as an evening charge RN at another hospital for 3 years since completing her BSN degree. She is excited about starting a new job but is apprehensive about the staff accepting her as a CNS. She wonders to herself, "Do I know enough to do this job?"

Kate, a classmate of Gloria's, has the same concerns. Kate has worked as a staff RN at the community hospital for 15 years before pursuing her dream of becoming a CNS. The director of nursing offered Kate a position as a CNS in the hospital following graduation. She's worried that her coworkers won't take her seriously in her new role. Gloria and Kate both recognize the importance of establishing credibility in their new roles.

Webster's Unabridged Dictionary (2001) defines credible as "1. capable of being believed; believable. 2. worthy of belief or confidence; trustworthy." Credibility requires clinical expertise, the thoughtful application of knowledge, and the demonstration of behaviors that create a reputation of trustworthiness. When Kouzes and Posner (1993) asked people to define credibility in behavioral terms, "the most frequent response was 'they do what they say they will do', 'they practice what they preach', 'they walk the talk', and 'their actions are consistent with their words'" (p. 47). The credibility foundation is built brick by brick. It is earned over time and sustained through hard work. A solid foundation of personal credibility is necessary for the CNS to generate confidence, gain commitment from others, and achieve desired patient outcomes or organizational goals and objectives.

Establishing Credible Relationships

Gloria is excited about her new job at the medical center but isn't sure where to start. To facilitate her transition (integration) to the CNS role, Gloria's supervisor asked Helen, an experienced CNS at the medical center, to be Gloria's "buddy." In addition, Gloria's supervisor has developed a structured orientation plan for her. Whether new or experienced, the CNS needs the time and opportunity to become acquainted with the organizational structure, mission, policies, and procedures of the institution. Also included in Gloria's orientation are appointments with key individuals. It will be important for Gloria to establish a credible relationship with the formal and informal leaders in the organization to accomplish the desired patient care outcomes. The meetings will be a first step by providing Gloria with an opportunity to understand each person's responsibilities and explain her role as a CNS and how she can be a valuable resource. These individuals may vary based on departmental structure and specific job description and responsibilities.

- Nursing administrators
- Physicians
- Nurse managers/assistant nurse managers
- Unit charge nurses, preceptors
- Administrative supervisors
- Interdisciplinary team members: pharmacist, chaplain, dietician, therapists
- CNS colleagues
- Nurse educators
- Quality Improvement/Quality Assurance staff
- Data analysts

Prior to the appointments, Helen helped Gloria understand the "lay of the land" in the organization: the administrative reporting structure, departmental relationships, and who to call. Helen commented that one of the most difficult things when she started her job was deciphering the organizational process for implementing practice changes. She shared the following example with Gloria. One of the first practices in need of change was implementation of the evidence-based recommendations for safe handling of hazardous drugs. At the suggestion of her buddy, she initially visited with the safety officer; directors of pharmacy, environmental services, and central supply; and nurse managers of oncology and critical care. She received support for the practice change but also received differing opinions of the sequence of steps necessary for implementation and whether final approval belonged to the safety officer, the director of nursing, or the nursing practice committee. Instead of trying to determine the process herself, she invited the key individuals to a meeting and together they identified the necessary changes, the sequence for implementation, and who had final approval. Helen commented that because of her approach she felt she had begun to gain the trust of several leaders in the organization.

From Staff Nurse Credible to Expert Credible: Dealing With Challengers

Despite her years of experience as an RN prior to becoming a CNS, Kate found herself unprepared for her feelings of inadequacy when being questioned by staff about a patient care issue outside her area of expertise. Now that she was the specialist, the staff teasingly commented she should know everything. Kate admitted she thought she should know the answer because a CNS is the expert. After a particularly difficult week, Kate began to wonder if she really belonged in this position. Fortunately, Kate shared her doubts with her supervisor, who reassured her that these feelings are normal, especially in a new role or a new job. She also told Kate the good news is the longer she stays in her CNS role and develops more expertise and knowledge, the less often she will experience these feelings of doubt and inadequacy.

The term *impostor phenomenon* has been used throughout psychology and sociology literature to describe individuals who feel as if they are impostors in their chosen profession. Often, it is a transient experience associated with specific situations such as starting a new job or moving into a new role (Harvey & Katz, 1985). Clinical symptoms associated with this phenomenon are generalized anxiety, lack of self-confidence, depression, and frustration related to an inability to meet a self-imposed standard of achievement (Clance & Imes, 1978). Arena and Page (1992) believe that a form of the impostor phenomenon is inherent in the CNS role. It is characterized by feelings of inadequacy and of constantly being tested, no matter how confident or self-secure the CNS feels. Questioning whether she or he belongs in the position may become all-encompassing and should be expected with a new role. These feelings may resurface when a change occurs in the role. If these symptoms extend into the CNS's personal life, the person may be experiencing the full effects of the phenomenon.

To help ease the feelings of doubt, Kate and her supervisor identified several strategies she can implement:

- First, find a CNS mentor with whom she can share her feelings and who will help Kate reestablish her self-confidence.
- Identify supportive colleagues at work who are willing to share their knowledge and expertise.
- Continue to provide direct patient care on a regular basis to maintain and strengthen clinical skills and develop clinical competence in weak areas.
- Develop a personal library by gathering and maintaining current information on relevant clinical topics. Kate can use the information to answer clinical questions from staff or post copies of journal articles pertinent to the unit's patient population.

■ Name a difference she has made to a patient, family, staff member, or colleague every day.

Kate's first step was to contact Brenda, a CNS at another hospital in town. Brenda, a CNS for 5 years, was delighted when Kate asked for her help and guidance. She shared with Kate her initial challenge of working with a nurse manager who felt threatened by her involvement and therefore didn't want any CNS help on the unit. Kate admitted she was grateful that that hadn't been a problem for her, but was intrigued to learn how Brenda dealt with this challenge. Brenda shared that she had taken the advice of her mentor, who suggested she focus on the units where her help was wanted, not stress over the manager who didn't understand the CNS role. Within a year, the skeptical nurse manager asked Brenda for her help. She had heard from several other nurse managers that Brenda had been helpful in working with staff to identify appropriate solutions to specific clinical practice issues and had been a valuable clinical role model and mentor for new nurses on their areas.

Demonstrating Credibility

After several months, Brenda invited Kate to attend a quarterly CNS networking meeting attended by CNSs from surrounding communities. At the meeting, Kate saw Gloria and asked how she was enjoying her new job. Gloria shared her struggles with being new in an organization: getting acquainted with key individuals, learning the organization structure, and gaining the trust of the nursing staff. Kate commented that her struggles have surprised her. She thought the transition to CNS would be easy, as she was familiar with the organization and the nursing staff. She didn't expect to be questioned about her knowledge and challenged about ulterior motives, such as being after the nurse manager's job.

Brenda introduced Kate and Gloria and asked the other CNSs to share a strategy or personal example of what they did as new CNSs to gain the confidence of others and gain credibility. The CNSs in attendance were eager to share their suggestions, because as one nurse commented, "We've all been there at least once." Suggested strategies include:

■ Schedule time for direct patient care and don't cancel. Working as staff and caring for patients in difficult situations provide an opportunity to prove your skills as a nurse and demonstrate your value as a useful resource.
■ Work an off shift periodically to demonstrate competence, serve as a role model, and provide opportunity for interaction and problem solving with evening and night staff. It also allows the CNS to observe actual implementation of nursing processes and procedures.
■ Attend shift report and team meetings and/or conduct patient-centered rounds, focusing on patient and family needs. Discuss and problem-solve issues identified during report or rounds with the nursing staff.
■ Participate in staff meetings and offer to present a short educational program on a topic identified through a needs assessment.
■ Offer to provide clinical expertise during a root cause analysis process or investigation of an unexpected patient outcome.

- Assist nurse educators or nurse managers with staff competencies or a hospital-wide education day.
- Write a brief article on a relevant clinical topic for a nursing unit or nursing department newsletter.

One strategy that received resounding agreement was the importance of maintaining a regular presence on the nursing areas. This also allows the CNS to promote her or his area of expertise. Joan shared her experience to illustrate this point. As a CNS with extensive pain management experience, Joan struggled with getting the staff to utilize her expertise. One day during patient rounds, Joan identified a patient with inadequate postoperative pain control despite the efforts of the nursing staff. During her patient interview and assessment, Joan discovered the patient had been taking a long-acting opioid for the past year due to a chronic pain condition. On admission, the long-acting opioid had not been continued, and the amount of IV analgesic the patient was receiving for post-op pain control was less than the patient had been taking preoperatively, accounting for the inadequate pain management. Joan shared her findings and recommendations with the staff nurse and the physician. During rounds the next day, the patient told Joan his pain was much better and he had been able to get some sleep during the night. Seeing Joan on the unit, a staff nurse asked her to see another patient about pain management. Several days later, Joan also received a consult request from the physician to see a patient for pain control suggestions. Joan firmly believes her constant visibility made the difference in laying the foundation for establishing her credibility as a CNS.

Credibility is about being believed, being competent, and being trustworthy. It provides the foundation for the CNS to generate confidence, gain commitment from others, and achieve desired patient outcomes or organizational goals and objectives. Credibility does make a difference.

References

Arena, D. M., & Page, N. E. (1992). The imposter phenomenon in the clinical nurse specialist role. *Image: Journal of Nursing Scholarship, 24*(2), 121–125.

Clance, P. R., & Imes, S. A. (1978). The imposter phenomenon in high achieving women: Dynamics and therapeutic intervention. *Psychotherapy: Theory, Research and Practice, 15*(3), 241–246.

Harvey, J. C., & Katz, C. (1985). *If I'm so successful, why do I feel like a fake? The imposter phenomenon.* New York: St. Martin's Press.

Kouzes, J. M., & Posner, B. Z. (1993). *Credibility: How leaders gain and lose it, why people demand it.* San Francisco: Jossey-Bass Publishers.

Webster's Unabridged Dictionary (2nd ed.). (2001). New York: Random House.

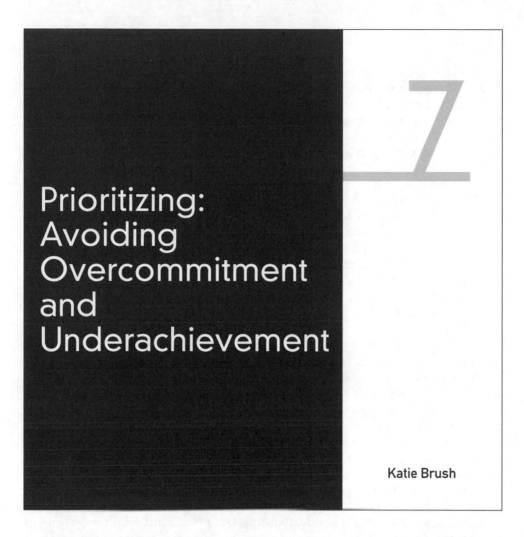

Prioritizing: Avoiding Overcommitment and Underachievement

7

Katie Brush

Welcome to a new role. Welcome to the world of the clinical nurse specialist (CNS). Welcome to the world of time management. Time management is essential to avoiding overcommitment, which is the slippery slope toward underachievement. The first year of CNS practice can be frustrating due to learning to juggle multiple competing demands and divergent responsibilities. Hopefully, this chapter will give you some tips on achieving balance and avoiding the pitfalls of this new practice.

A new CNS is presented with many opportunities to make a difference, such as introducing evidence-based practice, leading performance improvement, and updating procedures—initiatives aimed at improving patient care and outcomes. A new CNS is eager to become involved and demonstrate new skills. In the beginning, it may seem as though there is a massive amount of work to do. With so many opportunities, a novice CNS is vulnerable to overcommitment; thus, time management becomes critical from the very beginning. Most new CNSs worked as staff nurses before going to graduate school. Staff nurse work has rather defined boundaries—the schedule is fixed, days and times determined, the patient assignment is clear, and when the shift is over, a staff nurse goes home. Not so for the CNS. A typical new CNS is not well prepared to manage multiple competing demands at the system level. Sure, graduate school had numerous deadlines, and meeting the demands of multiple assignments may have been challenging; however, the difference is that now *you*, the CNS, participate in determining the assignment. Many new CNSs underestimate the amount of time and energy needed to develop, implement, evaluate, revise, monitor, and continuously support unit level or system level projects. Avoid believing you can leap tall buildings in a single bound. It's not true for anyone, but for a novice it is a sure way to fail.

There will always be colleagues, staff, and bosses ready to fill the plate of the new CNS. It is a great honor for the new CNS to be trusted enough to be asked to take on important projects. Be cautious: Start small. Select projects where the time to completion is delimited and the chance of success is high. Too many projects, projects that are complex, or projects that may take months or years to complete will not give a new CNS the gratification and confidence that success builds. Despite coursework, no matter how helpful, role-related culture shock is present from the moment you enter the work world as a new CNS. Before saying yes to an assignment, ask yourself: Am I up to this challenge? Is this the best project for me at this time? Can I succeed? Remember to start small and build a record of successes.

The boss can help you prioritize. Discuss your goals with the boss, and determine the boss's goals for you. The negotiation process between the two of you should take into account your level of experience. If the boss has never worked with a CNS, or worked with CNSs in roles not including competencies in the three spheres—patient, nurses/nursing practice, and system—you may also need to negotiate the focus of your role. CNSs eager to please may be inclined to take on any project assigned by the boss. Negotiate! Be prepared to discuss how the new project fits into your current priorities. Ask the boss: What would you like me to give up in order to take this on? Asked respectfully in the context of prioritizing your work, it is not insubordination. Prioritizing with the boss helps you control your workload. Discuss current projects and assignments, progress toward completion, and rationale for ongoing involvement. The boss may have an entirely different idea. Listen to the boss's viewpoint. The ability to compromise and listen to each other is essential. But don't negotiate away all the things you enjoy. The job will become drudgery unless you are able to keep some things that you value most in your list of priorities. For example, if you enjoy making rounds in the intensive care unit to "case find" patient problems, don't eliminate this completely to take on a major project that will remove you from the unit for months. Compromise! You might reduce your rounds from daily to three times a week and ask for an assistant or co-chair for the project.

The Nursing Staff

As a new CNS, you must meet the staff—nurses, therapists, clerks, housekeepers, and others who work in your specialty area. Learn their names, years of experience, and type of assignments they prefer. Observe practice and consider spending time orienting to the staff nurse role in the specialty setting. Remind staff that you will not be very effective in helping them with patient care if you don't understand patient care in the unit. Be clear that you are not orienting so you can fill in for vacations, lunch assignments, or unanticipated absences. You are learning the role so you can appreciate their perspective and understand their challenges and opportunities. Orientation is time limited. Let the staff know the time—a couple of weeks should be adequate to learn the staff nurse role. Depending on your familiarity with the unit or type of care setting, more or less time for orientation may be needed.

While orienting, ask the staff about things they would change if they could. Listen to what issues each staff member identifies as problems. Keep a list, and review it for similarities among staff members. Create categories of ideas that you may want to address in the future. Prioritize the ideas. Start small. Nothing breeds success like fixing a relatively simple problem that has irritated staff for a prolonged time. It may be a problem that you would never have considered until the staff pointed it out. You will win the staff's trust when you successfully address their problems.

Colleagues

Colleagues can be your best allies. They can help you sort out some of your big and small questions. Learn from others' experiences and value stories for the lessons they teach. Spend time with other junior colleagues and see how they are managing. Keep your eyes and ears open. Watch for habits that some colleagues may have developed that you want to avoid, such as spending late nights working on projects or being involved in so many things that they are ineffective. Notice how others manage time well and make respected contributions. Try to emulate the good work habits and avoid the pitfalls. A successful CNS has often spent years learning to stay focused, manage time, prioritize projects, and avoid overcommitment. Ask experienced CNSs to share secrets to prioritizing tasks and managing time.

Flying Under the Radar

Role success means being effective. You cannot be effective if you are stretched too thin. A new CNS should ascribe to the notion of "flying under the radar," or, in other words, keeping a low profile. Don't volunteer for every committee, program, project, and work group. Be selective. Spend most of your time listening. Give yourself time to learn the organizational culture. Begin by focusing your efforts on staff and patient care. There will be pressure to join in the projects involving the global arena. Listen to the concerns, but don't offer your time. Learn the politics. You are a "can do" professional, but avoid the desire to do everything for everyone.

Your arrival has been eagerly awaited and productivity anticipated. Most likely, many individuals will have preconceived ideas of your role and have formulated goals. Others may want to assign projects and committee work to you. In a meeting with a group of your peers, or with any group who is interested in a new endeavor, you do *not* need to jump in—don't be the first to volunteer. Suffer through the uncomfortable silences that arise in the group and wait for a more experienced person to volunteer. You are eager to please and prove your abilities, but this is a sure way to become overcommitted and ineffective. If the project is complex, you may feel overwhelmed. This feeling is a good indication that the project is something you should avoid. If it becomes necessary to take on the new project, ask for another, more senior CNS to work with you.

It is an honor to be asked to contribute. The feeling of being needed is gratifying. The idea that your opinion is important can be terrifying and thrilling at the same time. Set priorities that will most benefit your cohort of patients, whether through the staff or the system. Work on a few value-added projects. Choose opportunities that will have the greatest effect on improvement in patient care in your area(s).

Carve out a niche in your area of expertise within your first years of practice by carefully selecting problems and projects that will build your reputation of success. Become the "go to" person for one or two patient care issues. Soon you will be receiving requests to consult on problems related to your niche specialty focus, which will give you more insight into the organization. The more knowledge you gain about your specialty area within the organization, the more you will be able to contribute.

Time Management

Maybe you are a great planner, scheduler, or finisher, or you may have great coordination skills. If this is true of you, keep it up! If not, find ways to be better organized. The job of a CNS can become a real time management nightmare. Poor time planning by CNSs is perhaps one of the worst problems in practice. It is a source of stress, a never-ending battle of trying to catch up. The worse your time management and planning skills are, the further behind you can fall.

It is very easy to become overwhelmed when you think of all of the things that need to be done. When considering things that should be dealt with, think about what must be done immediately, what needs to be done in the near future, and what can be put into the timeline of things to do. Make a list. If you have difficulty sorting out what needs to be completed by when, think about the tasks from a chi square perspective: high importance, low importance, urgent, non urgent. Visuals such as calendars, timelines, and color-coded notes are an asset to most people. Use any method that helps you sort and prioritize—paper checklists, reminder lists on the computer, a PDA device. Time management is only as good as your ability to stick to it.

Life/Work Balance

With all of the new opportunities and challenges, a new CNS can be tempted to work long hours, but long days can leave you exhausted and ultimately undermine your ability to achieve. Long hours at work can strain personal relationships, cause loss of enjoyable activities, and create additional stress both at home and at work.

A new CNS is particularly vulnerable to diving into more and more work and losing balance. Use time management strategies and goal setting to leave work at work when you walk out the door. Maintain the things in life that bring you pleasure. Set personal priorities to avoid being consumed by work. Do not lose your identity so much that the center of your being is focused on your CNS role.

Personal and professional priorities should be balanced to avoid feeling overwhelmed. Make balance in all things your mantra. Make a list of your priorities. Post the list in your office within view. When you are tempted to take on an additional project, read the list, remember why you made it, and ask, "Is this value added to my patient population, the staff, the system that supports the staff, and to me professionally? What else is on my plate? Can it wait? Can other projects be put on hold? Does it conflict with my personal goals?" (Covey, 1989, p. 106).

Tipping Point

The tasks and projects can be overwhelming. Patient care takes priority and can change your calendar in a moment. Meetings can take up much of your time. In the novice phase, if you have more than three to four meetings a week, you've probably gone too far. If these meetings take time away from focusing on the patients and staff, again, you have lost the battle with time management. You will have reached the tipping point—the "moment of critical mass, the threshold, the boiling point" (Gladwell, 2000, p. 12). Make appointments with yourself to revise your priorities, revisit timelines, and negotiate duties. Reorganize, re-prioritize, and reenergize.

Lessons Learned

Let's examine the tale of two CNSs. The first CNS manages her time by outlining projects, addressing quantity of work, and making appointments for self time—time to think and work alone. She is able to keep current with research, is known for bringing evidence to the bedside, and has excellent outcomes within the three spheres. She meets her outbound train on time every day and doesn't take work home. She maintains her interests and relationships.

The second CNS is in her first CNS job. She was pleased and honored when asked to be involved in things. She makes patient care a priority even though her assigned units of coverage have grown from 1 to 9. She takes on most everything requested by staff in her units and is involved in multiple committees that all impact patient care in her specialty. She feels it is her responsibility to be the voice for nursing in the specialty area. She has no mentors. She is known for being late and turning in work late—which is quite different from graduate school, where she was envied by other students for being well prepared for class and never handing in an assignment late. She works 10 to 12 hour days and regularly takes work home. Her friends complain that they never see her and stop inviting her to parties and events. She thinks that she has learned a lot and has been a successful CNS.

The novice CNS above was me. A year after changing jobs, I was chatting with a staff nurse in one of the units I covered, and when I mentioned that I often thought of the nurses in that unit, she replied, "I don't know why, you were never there." Ouch!! Lesson learned. It took a life-changing experience to make me see that I was overwhelmed and achieving little. I learned to balance my life and work—to be more like the first CNS example and less like the second.

Although I am tempted to overcommit, I have gotten better about asking for information before jumping in. I inquire about estimated time needed for the project, extent of the project, and possible benefits for patients and staff in my areas of responsibility. I look at what else is *on my plate*. I go through my calendar and see how much time I am spending out of my clinical area. If the project is more than I can afford to do, I go back to what my priorities are. I use the list method, with due dates, and committee responsibilities. I try to keep current with tasks and deadlines.

I have been involved in the Critical Care Committee (CCC) since I began my "new" job 10 years ago. About 5 years ago, I was appointed to be the first nurse co-chair of the committee. There is enormous responsibility and practice throughout our facility through the work of the CCC. Prior to changing to a prioritization style of work, I put the agenda together, took the minutes and typed them, and implemented all the organizational-level practice changes within critical care. Because of this co-chair position, I was constantly asked to do more and more with critical care and related issues. I always said yes. My life-changing experience helped me change my approach to the CCC. I created co-chairs and requested that they take over the agenda and the minutes and make appropriate follow-ups to achieve project completion. I still work on projects for the CCC but no longer carry the full burden. The workload of this committee is much more balanced now.

I am more willing to refer individuals to my other CNS colleagues with expertise in the problem being presented. I no longer volunteer to take on everything. I elicit the help of my manager in looking at my commitments and offers of projects. As a result, I usually work about 9 hours a day. I leave on time and feel guilt free to do the personal things. I enjoy spending my time sailing, meeting with friends, and traveling. I take vacations! I have finally realized that I am not indispensable. I understand that highly successful people say no all the time, and that successful people view the decision to say no as equally acceptable as the decision to say yes.

Conclusion

The shortest full sentence in the English language is "No." Remember it, as it will serve you well.

References

Covey, S. R. (1989). *The seven habits of highly effective people; Restoring the character ethic*. New York: Simon and Schuster.
Gladwell, M. (2000). *The tipping point*. Boston: Little, Brown, and Company.

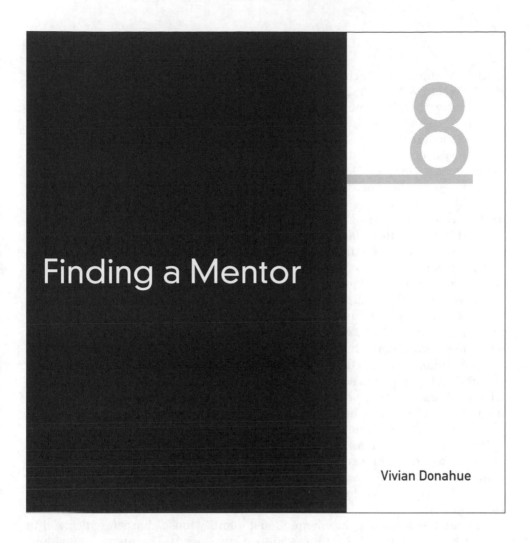

Finding a Mentor

8

Vivian Donahue

A wise man learns by the experiences of others.
An ordinary man learns by his own experience.
A fool learns by nobody's experience.

—*Anonymous*

This chapter is titled "Finding a Mentor." Your first thought might be simple enough. The clinical nurse specialist (CNS) is an advanced practice nurse who has extensive knowledge and experience in respective specialties. One might identify a CNS who has similar interests and areas of expertise and seek him or her out as a mentor. But before you embark on your journey to find a mentor, you must first consider: What does a mentor do, and what am I hoping to achieve with this relationship?

Much of the literature describes the mentoring experiences in the business world, where the concept of mentoring had its early beginnings. The term *mentor* was first introduced in Homer's *Odyssey* and has long been established in the business world but appears to have entered the nursing profession in the 1970s. "The new mentorship initiative is an emerging paradigm in which we have an unprecedented opportunity to strengthen our identity and create new models of support and achievement in our schools, workplaces, and the profession" (Greene & Puetzer, 2002, p. 64).

Clearly the role of mentor has taken on significant importance in both our professional and personal lives. To begin a mentoring relationship we must first answer the question, what does a mentor do? There are numerous definitions, but the concept of mentor continues to evolve. As it evolves, the descriptions become more complex. Descriptions involve characteristics of the relationship, the mentee, and, the mentor.

Within the numerous definitions lies some description of the individuals involved in mentoring. Most would identify a distinct set of characteristics. Roemer (2002) states that "the concept of mentoring includes two elements: professional assistance, in the form of coaching and access to opportunity, and psychosocial support" (p. 57). Greene and Puetzer (2002) describe the mentoring initiative as one that provides an opportunity to strengthen our identity and create new models of support and achievement within the profession. A mentor has also been described as "someone who is a trusted advisor, teacher and wise person" (McKinley, 2004, p. 206). "Mentors are often those individuals who possess the qualities that others want to emulate" (Kanaskie, 2006, p. 248).

A common thread in the literature describing mentorships includes professional development and social support. Many descriptions of a mentor include a list of characteristics. A discussion of these characteristics may illuminate the mentoring process most effectively. Characteristics ascribed to mentors include patience, enthusiasm, knowledge, sense of humor, and respect (Kanaskie, 2006, p. 249). Roles of mentors include teacher, advisor, and good listener. The list will vary based on the needs of the mentee. In conjunction with the suggested characteristics, there are techniques both formal and informal utilized by the most effective mentors to develop and support the mentees in their professional growth.

In seeking a mentor, the mentee must identify those characteristics within that individual that will meet one's professional needs. The mentee must also identify a mentor with whom one is capable of sustaining a long-term relationship. Ideally a mentee should reflect on and identify personal strengths, weaknesses, and needs prior to seeking out a mentor.

The terms *teaching, coaching, role modeling,* and *precepting* are often used interchangeably with *mentoring.* Role modeling, coaching, and teaching are all tools that can be utilized by a mentor to promote professional development and socialization of the mentee. Each of these tools plays a role in the mentoring process but is not alone sufficient in describing a mentor. "We are all role models, whether we like it or not. Our actions, words, body language, and behavior are always being observed by others" (Girard, 2006, p. 13). All mentors are role models, but not all role models are capable of mentoring. The term *preceptor* is often used interchangeably with *mentor* although there are distinctions. A preceptor implies a short-term relationship, often assigned formally for educational purposes, and is often involved in the evaluative process.

The term *mentor* implies a long-term relationship, most often informally initiated based on the mentee's needs. A mentor continues to promote professional growth throughout the mentee's career (Fawcett, 2002). The duration of the mentoring experience cannot be defined but instead is one focused on development of independent practice on the part of the mentee (Ihlenfeld, 2005).

As with all developmental roles within the nursing profession, this relationship can be based on the principles of Pat Benner's (2001) *novice to expert* approach. In this scenario the mentor would be practicing at the expert level, and the mentee would be a novice in the role. Role development would continue until a mutually agreed upon level of practice had been achieved. The relationship may become a lifetime commitment.

The characteristics most often ascribed to mentors help create an environment conducive to developing a long-term relationship. Patience is needed to provide the mentee an opportunity to learn. Support and guidance are offered to help the mentee learn new tasks and to create an environment of success. Enthusiasm encourages the mentee to seek out new experiences and to avoid complacency (Fawcett, 2002). Knowledge is shared between the mentor and the mentee. Knowing one's weakness allows the mentor to seek advice from experts and gain insight from the mentoring experience.

Mentoring involves mutual respect and reflection. Both mentor and mentee must be able to reflect objectively on their practice. This is a synergistic relationship meant to promote professional development for both the mentee and the mentor. Mentoring impacts the mentor, the mentee, and the organization. "The rewards for the mentee include advice and guidance on how to succeed within the unit and organization" (McKinley, 2004). Mentors are empowered by their potential to help another person, and both the mentor and the mentee are giving back to the organization and the profession (McKinley, 2004, p. 209). Positive outcomes of the mentoring experience include improved retention and promoting professionalism.

Mentoring can be described as a process. McKinley (2004) speaks to a three-step process including reflecting, reframing, and resolving. "Reflecting is the creation of the relationship. Reframing is making the connection with the organization or unit. Resolving is empowering the individual to problem solve and identify progress toward positive outcomes" (p. 209).

Many co-factors may affect one's ability to develop a mentoring relationship. Factors may include gender, age, socioeconomic status, and personality (Roemer, 2002, p. 58). Many of these co-factors continue to be of ongoing interest to researchers. The literature is varied in its interpretation of these factors. The varied interpretation of factors suggests that further research is needed to identify the impact of these factors on the role of mentor.

Mentoring provides a unique opportunity for the CNS as both a mentor and a mentee. France (2006) states that "clinical coaching and the mentor-protégé relationship in the clinical setting create an environment for learning, collegiality, and self-confidence in the role" (p. 97). Role socialization has been clearly identified as an integral component of retention. Mentoring provides an opportunity to support our colleagues and promote socialization. In terms of definitions alone we speak of identifying unit and organizational idiosyncrasies and assisting the mentee in gaining an understanding of these idiosyncrasies. This understanding promotes socialization and ultimately self-confidence in the new CNS.

As there are individual characteristics descriptive of a positive mentor, there are also characteristics that would not promote an effective mentor–mentee relationship. Individuals who lack knowledge in communication skills and listening would not be effective mentors. A mentor must recognize that he or she is a role model and teacher. As such, one must be able to advocate for the mentee and promote a positive learning experience. Individuals who lack a positive outlook may not be able to provide this experience. Darling (1985) describes toxic mentors and suggests they fall into four categories: avoiders, dumpers, blockers, and destroyers or criticizers. We have all encountered individuals who exhibit one or more of these characteristics. Individuals who exhibit such behaviors would be excluded as ideal mentors.

An individual may choose to identify with one individual as a mentor or several individuals throughout his or her career. This process may evolve as the CNS develops. At varying times throughout his or her career, needs may need to be reassessed. Professional growth continues throughout one's career and as new opportunities present themselves. A mentor may or may not be someone within the role of CNS. The role of a CNS is expansive; the behavior or skill one chooses to emulate may be found in other nursing roles.

Now that we have identified the characteristics of a mentor, it may be helpful to identify why one would choose to seek out a mentor. First we may examine the role of the mentee. Feeling anxious and unsure of oneself is a natural sensation when undertaking a new endeavor. There are many benefits for the mentee once a mentor–mentee relationship has developed. One benefit is the process of becoming embedded within the organization. This process is promoted through socialization, guidance in practice, and reassurances offered by the mentor. Each of these gains in turn promotes commitment to the organization and the profession. A process of enculturing develops and the mentee begins to grow and develop until he or she too becomes a mentor.

Mentoring relationships help both the mentor and the mentee develop a better understanding of each other's values and practices. Generational differences often create challenges to understanding each other's values. Developing a trusting relationship allows the participants to communicate in such a way that they begin to understand each other's belief systems and values.

A mentee is less likely to experience burnout and is more likely to feel rewarded in a career. A mentee is more likely to become a mentor as he or she matures in a career, thereby creating a positive cycle within the profession. And finally, a mentee is more likely to advance in a professional career.

A mentor also benefits from this relationship. The mentor develops a better understanding of values and practices via the relationship with the mentee. Mentoring promotes growth and further practice development of the mentor. Some literature supports the theory that as the mentee becomes less dependent on the mentor, a more collegial relationship develops, creating a mutually supportive relationship.

There are also organizational benefits. Retention is improved. Professional commitment on behalf of the organization becomes apparent. The organizational support for professional practice promotes an environment that encourages teamwork. A positive, healthy work environment ensues. Mentoring provides an understanding of the mission and vision of an organization through discussion and clarification of the organization's values (McKinley, 2004, p. 208).

Mentoring is a means to promote the profession of nursing. Mentoring develops potential leaders within the organization and the profession (Kanaskie, 2006, p. 250). "Nursing exists in a very complex world. To successfully navigate in that world, nurses need to mentor each other. Without mentoring, nurses become burned out and lose the spark of commitment to the profession" (Scott, 2005, p. 52). Many authors suggest that informal mentoring (those relationships that develop due to a shared or common interest) occurs frequently and spontaneously in nursing. It is this kind of ongoing commitment to the profession that will move nursing forward into the future.

Mentoring provides a structure for growth, professional satisfaction, and the ability to give back to colleagues and the profession. Mentors come in many forms. My first mentor was the nurse manager on the unit where I began my career. She was an incredibly intelligent, insightful, and giving nurse. Her commitment to the staff and the nursing profession was evident in every aspect of her practice. Nurse S provided positive reinforcement to promote my strengths, helped me identify those areas for potential improvement, and saw professional commitment in my practice. Nurse S provided me with recommendations for a clinical recognition program to develop my practice and foster my self-confidence. She encouraged me to identify and speak to my career goals. When she discovered I had an interest in critical care nursing, she recommended me to her colleague who was the nurse manager of the medical intensive care unit. Without her encouragement and support I would not be a critical care CNS with over 25 years of critical care experience.

Nurse S was the first mentor in my career, but throughout my career I have identified those individuals whose qualities I have valued most and have sought their expertise and guidance. At every stage of my career, my needs have varied. While pursuing my master's degree in nursing I had the opportunity to experience the role with CNSs in varied settings. I am also fortunate to be able to practice in my role as a CNS in an organization that supports the role. There are approximately 50 CNSs in the organization, and we all seek the guidance of our colleagues, as each has a unique area of expertise.

We are also committed to the CNS students who choose to experience their clinical practicum within our institution. The ability to apply our knowledge and share our expertise promotes our own professional development as well as that of the students. With organizational support the CNSs are able to foster a mentoring environment.

This journey began with the identification of two concepts in need of clarification. The first concept identified was the need to clearly articulate a definition of the term *mentor*. The second concept involved creating an appreciation for the mentor–mentee relationship. Several definitions were offered, all with common denominators. Characteristics of a mentor were identified. The mutually beneficial relationship of mentor–mentee was explored. And finally, the benefit incurred by the organization and the unit itself was discussed.

We are finally prepared to discuss how to find a mentor. Perhaps an algorithmic approach might be best (see Table 8.1). First the mentee must reflect on one's practice. Second, consideration must be given to which skills or practice the mentee would like to emulate. An individual with similar values, goals, and practice must be willing to engage in and commit to the mentor–mentee relationship. And finally, a mutually rewarding, long-lasting relationship must be developed between the two individuals. If this can be accomplished, one will have successfully found a mentor.

In conclusion, mentoring promotes potential growth in the mentee and the mentor, and at the unit or organizational level. A commitment must be made to

8.1 Finding a Mentor

Reflective practice

↓

Identification of skills/practice mentee wishes to emulate

↓

Mentor with similar values/goals engages in and commits to relationship

↓

Mutually rewarding, long-term relationship develops

↓

Professional growth and development are supported

↓

Nursing profession advances toward a rewarding future

the process for all involved for mentoring to be successful. Once committed to the process, all participants will benefit from the experience, and the nursing profession will continue to grow and develop.

References

Benner, P. (2001). *From novice to expert: Excellence and power in clinical nursing practice.* Menlo Park, CA: Addison-Wesley.

Darling, L. A. (1985). What to do about toxic mentors. *Journal of Nursing Administration, 15*(5), 43–44.

Fawcett, D. L. (2002). Mentoring: What it is and how to make it work (Research/Education). *Association of Operating Room Nurses, 75*(5), 950–954.

France, N.E.M. (2006). Socializing clinical nurse specialist students for practice. *Clinical Nurse Specialist, 20*(2), 97–99.

Girard, N. J. (2006). Like it or not you are a role model. *Association of Operating Room Nurses, 84*(1), 13–15.

Greene, M. T., & Puetzer, M. (2002). The value of mentoring: A strategic approach to retention and recruitment. *Journal of Nursing Care Quality, 17*(1), 63–70.

Ihlenfeld, J. T. (2005). Hiring and mentoring graduate nurses in the intensive care unit. *Dimensions of Critical Care Nursing, 24*(4), 175–178.

Kanaskie, M. L. (2006). Mentoring: A staff retention tool. *Critical Care Nursing Quarterly, 29*(3), 248–252.

McKinley, M. G. (2004). Mentoring matters: Creating, connecting, empowering. *AACN Clinical Issues, 15*(2), 205–214.

Roemer, L. (2002). Women CEOs in health care: Did they have mentors? *Health Care Management Review, 27*(4), 57–67.

Scott, E. S. (2005). Peer-to-peer mentoring teaching collegiality. *Nurse Educator, 30*(2), 52–56.

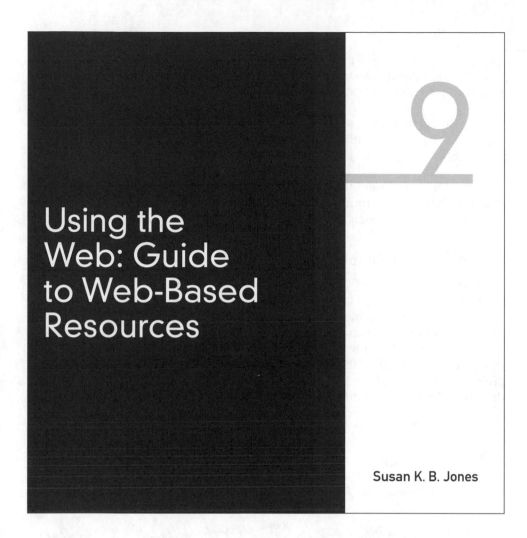

Using the Web: Guide to Web-Based Resources

Susan K. B. Jones

"It is the clinical nurse specialist (CNS) who works within the healthcare system to bridge the gap between what is known through research and what is done in the practice setting. As a consequence, the role played by CNSs will only grow in value over the next two decades. The overall safety of the healthcare delivery system and the patients entrusted to our care are being enhanced daily by the work of the CNS" (Goudreau et al., 2007). These responsibilities require that CNSs stay abreast of changing practice trends for the populations of patients with which they work. This means that the CNSs must stay connected to all of the sources of information that have the potential to impact their practice, their patients, and the organizations with which they work.

Staying connected includes using the internet. CNSs use the internet to remain connected to professional organizations, to search and find the best evidence that influences the way care is provided to patients and families, and to stay connected to national and international organizations conducting research and setting standards of practice for their patient populations. The importance of professional organizations and networking is addressed later in this toolkit. The focus of this section is the multiple ways that a CNS can use Web-based resources to provide and support quality patient care.

Although these resources could be organized in a variety of ways, for the purposes of this chapter they will be organized by:

- Global resources as they relate to evidence-based practice,
- Resources that influence organizational decisions, and
- Specialty patient population resources.

By no means should this be considered an exhaustive list of resources, but it should provide a beginning framework of the types of resources available for you and the professionals and patients with whom you work.

Organizational Resources

Irrespective of the CNS's population specialty, national groups influence the care of those patients. Figure 9.1 (Gelinas, 2007) represents some of the national policy-making groups and specialty organizations that influence the way care is provided. It is incumbent upon CNSs to be aware of recommendations that are promoted by these organizations. Although it is beyond the scope of this text to include all of the electronic addresses for these organizations, a simple electronic search for these organizations will provide the appropriate addresses. A brief examination of each of these sites will assist in identifying tools

9.1 The Quality Choir: Multitude of activities confronting hospitals creates initiative overload.

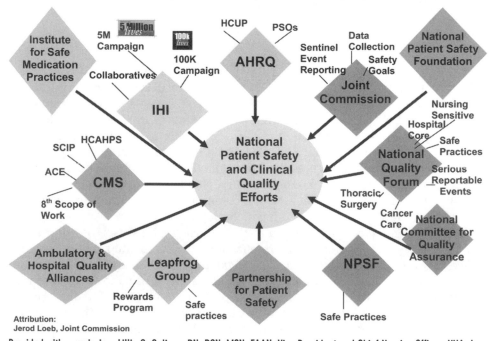

Attribution:
Jerod Loeb, Joint Commission

Provided with permission: Lillie S. Gelinas, RN, BSN, MSN, FAAN, Vice President and Chief Nursing Officer, VHA, Inc.

prepared to support the work of each group. For example, information found on the Institute for Healthcare Improvement (2007) Web site (http://ihi.org/ihi) includes information about the 100K Lives and 5 Million Lives campaigns. There are links to how-to kits for each of the initiatives addressed in these campaigns. This type of information is helpful in providing the background material for national initiatives in an easy-to-use format.

Evidence-Based Practice Resources

Resources for finding the evidence on which to base your practice are not necessarily as easy to come by. Staying abreast of the ever-changing research base upon which CNSs base practice decisions can be a full-time job. To remain successful in this arena, it is important to maximize your efforts. This means knowing the most helpful internet sites, identifying which (if any) databases you have access to through your organization or school, and developing a close working relationship with the librarians in both locations. In order to understand where to begin to look, it is important to understand the many different types of information available for review. Where you seek information will be determined by the type of information you are looking for. If you are looking for individual primary research articles, you will likely begin by searching one of the databases such as Pubmed (searches MEDLINE) or CINHAL. Electronic access to Pubmed (http://www.ncbi.nlm.nih.gov/sites/entrez) is available through the National Library of Medicine and the National Institutes of Health without subscription for access to the citation and the abstract for those articles. However, to access the full-text versions of the articles, you must either purchase the article directly from Pubmed or have access through a subscription. In order to search the CINHAL database, a subscription to a service is required; EBSCO host is the current provider of this service. Many hospitals have subscriptions to services that enable online searching and retrieval of research articles. If your organization does not have a subscription of this type, consider contacting a librarian at a local, publicly funded university to establish a relationship. Explore what the librarian might be able to do to help you access the databases to which the institution subscribes.

While these types of databases are helpful in finding primary research articles, many of the topics that are important to CNS practice have been broadly researched and have conflicting findings. When systematic reviews of the literature are available, the information helps ensure that practice decisions are made using the best information available, and decisions are not necessarily based on a single study. Helpful sites for determining whether a systematic review of the literature has been performed include sites from the Cochrane Collaboration Library, the Joanna Briggs Institute (JBI), and others found in Table 9.1. The Cochrane Collaboration performs systematic reviews of the literature on topics of effectiveness; access to the Cochrane Library is available in the United States by subscription only (Cochrane Collaboration, 2007). Check with your organization and/or your higher education libraries to determine whether you have access to this information.

The JBI Web site provides information based on systematic reviews of the literature as well, but these reviews go beyond reviews of effectiveness. The JBI

9.1 Useful Web Sites for Clinical Nurse Specialists

Web Site	URL
Pubmed	http://www.ncbi.nlm.nih.gov/sites/entrez
Cochrane Library	http://www.cochrane.org/
Joanna Briggs Institute (JBI)	http://www.joannabriggs.edu.au/about/home.php
Center for the Advancement of Evidence Based Practice at Arizona State University	http://nursing.asu.edu/caep/
Academic Center for Evidence Based Practice at the University of Texas Health Sciences Center San Antonio	http://www.acestar.uthscsa.edu/default.html
University of Iowa Hospitals and Clinics Evidence Based Practice & Research Utilization	http://www.uihealthcare.com/depts/nursing/rqom/evidencebasedpractice/index.html
Agency for Healthcare Research and Quality (AHRQ)	http://www.ahrq.gov/
Centers for Disease Control & Prevention (CDC)	http://www.cdc.gov/
National Guidelines Clearinghouse (NGC)	http://www.guideline.gov/
National Quality Measures Clearinghouse (NQMC)	http://www.qualitymeasures.ahrq.gov/
Registered Nurses Association of Ontario (RNAO)—Nursing Best Practice Guidelines	http://www.rnao.org/Page.asp?PageID=861&SiteNodeID=133
American Association of Critical Care Nurses—Clinical Practice	http://www.aacn.org
Oncology Nurses Society—Evidence Based Practice Toolkits	http://onsopcontent.ons.org/toolkits/evidence/
Hartford Institute for Geriatric Nursing	http://www.hartfordign.org/
Society of Critical Care Medicine	http://www.sccm.org

also provides reviews of studies based upon the feasibility, appropriateness, and meaningfulness of health care practices (Joanna Briggs Institute, 2007). Information from the JBI systematic reviews of the literature (SRL) is available in several formats; the two most popular are the systematic review of the literature and the Best Practice Information Sheets (BPIS). The full-text SRL provides detailed information including the search strategy and in-depth information about the articles themselves. The BPISs provide a synopsis of the information from the SRL in an easy-to-read format. Additionally, the BPIS contains recommendations for practice as well as suggestions for future research. Access to the complete systematic reviews is available through membership only; access to many of the BPISs on JBI is available without subscription through the JBI Web site.

Beyond being aware of and being able to find systematic reviews of the literature, CNSs use the internet to locate and learn about national and international guidelines for care. These clinical practice guidelines come from a variety of organizations and in several differing formats. Table 9.1 lists Web addresses that may be helpful in identifying clinical practice guidelines for different populations. Each site has a search option that may be helpful in narrowing the scope of interest. Other Web sites with valuable information for clinicians wishing to use evidence-based practice as a foundation for decision making include the Center for the Advancement of Evidence Based Practice at Arizona State University, the Academic Center for Evidence Based Practice at the University of Texas Health Sciences Center at San Antonio, and the University of Iowa Hospitals and Clinics Division for Evidence Based Practice (URLs for these sites are included in Table 9.1).

Specialty Resources

Specialty organizations have become increasingly influential in setting the standards for providing patient care. Some organizations provide free access to the information related to their specialty populations, while others require membership for access. This membership requirement is another reason involvement in a specialty organization can be very beneficial to the CNS. Table 9.1 includes some of the specialty organization Web sites that allow non-member access to the best-practice information impacting particular populations of interest. Organizations such as the Infusion Nursing Society and the Association of Perioperative Registered Nurses have a plethora of information that is available through membership. (Please do not be offended if your specialty organization is not included. As stated previously, many organizations require membership in order to access their resource information. Those Web sites were not included.)

Listservs

Another important Web-based resource for CNSs and organizations that employ them are the numerous Listservs available. These Web-based groups provide subscribers with an opportunity to be a part of discussions presented and responded to by professionals from across the health care community. These groups provide individuals the opportunity to pose questions to the group, to learn how to address unique practice problems, and to network with national and international leaders. Some of the Listservs that are available include the National Association of Clinical Nurse Specialists Listserv (NACNS-list-owner@mail-list.com), the CNS Listserv (cns-listserv-d@mail-list.com), Advance Nursing Practice (ANPACC@yahoogroups.com), and Pediatric Advance Practice Nursing (PICUAPN@yahoogroups.com).

The information included in this chapter is representative of information available to CNSs and the organizations with whom they work, but it is by no means an exhaustive compilation. The information represents a framework on which CNSs can build to use the ever-changing content that is available via the internet to guide the care they and their organizations provide.

References

Cochrane Collaboration. (2007). Access to Cochrane. Retrieved September 18, 2007, from http://www3.interscience.wiley.com/cgi-bin/mrwhome/106568753/AccessCochrane Library.html

Gelinas, L. S. (2007). National nursing leadership update: A focus on nursing care and clinical quality. Presented at VHA Oklahoma-Arkansas Joint CNO Meeting, on September 21, 2007.

Goudreau, K. A., Baldwin, K., Clark, A., Fulton, J., Lyon, B., Murray, T., et al. (2007). A vision of the future for clinical nurse specialists. Prepared by the National Association of Clinical Nurse Specialists. Retrieved September 21, 2007, from http://www.nacns.org/A_Vision_of_the_Future_for_Clinical_Nurse_Specialists_final_7%2025%2007.pdf

Institute for Healthcare Improvement. (2007). *Topics*. Retrieved September 20, 2007, from http://www.ihi.org/ihi/topics

Joanna Briggs Institute. (2007). *About the Institute*. Retrieved September 20, 2007, from http://www.joannabriggs.edu.au/about/about.php

Gaining
Momentum

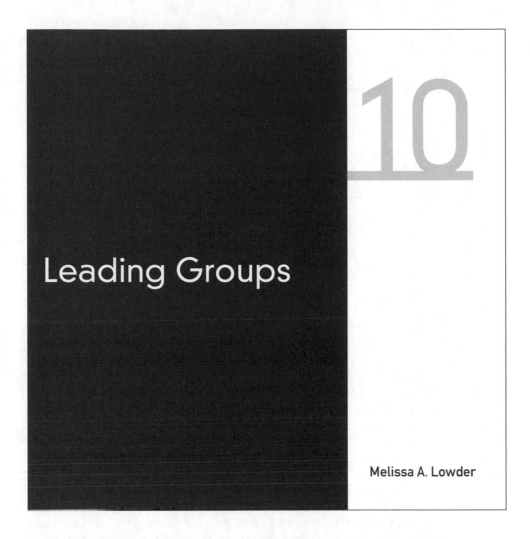

Leading Groups

Melissa A. Lowder

Sure, you've been a member of a committee before, but now you have been asked to chair a committee—to lead a group. Whether it's a new group or an existing one, who better than a clinical nurse specialist (CNS) to lead it? A core competency of CNS practice is to "lead nursing and multidisciplinary groups in implementing innovative patient care programs that address issues across the full continuum of care for different population groups and/or different specialties" (National Association of Clinical Nurse Specialists [NACNS], 2004, p. 36). CNSs have the education, experience, and clinical competency to lead groups for the purpose of patient care innovation or clinical program development, implementation, and evaluation.

Types of Groups

What type of group will you lead? Most often, groups are developed to disseminate information, seek opinions, and/or solve problems (Huber, 2000). Based on the purpose of the group, it may be structured in the organization as a task group (task force), a standing committee, a subcommittee, or an ad hoc group.

A task group consists of several persons who work together to accomplish a specific time-limited assignment (Sullivan & Decker, 2005). Groups of nurses working together to write a new policy on restraint care or design a patient education program are examples of task groups. In this type of group, members work independent of administrative leadership. With task groups, a CNS may bring the group together, clarify the charge and timeline, ensure that members have all needed resources, and then allow them to work independently, serving only as a facilitator.

Committees are created to address specific ongoing issues and may be single discipline or multidisciplinary. Committees exist as structural elements in the organization and may be created by bylaws or administrative units. In health care settings, standing committees usually involve several service areas or disciplines (Sullivan & Decker, 2005). An example of a standing committee would be a Patient Safety Committee that is responsible for monitoring and improving patient safety. Committees are very common in organizations and require strong leadership for efficient operations and targeted outcomes.

An ad hoc group or committee is designed to address a specific immediate need. Like a task force, it is a temporary group that functions within a specific time frame. Some ad hoc committees are formed as a subcommittee of a larger committee and charged with addressing one or two interrelated topics that are under the responsibility of a larger committee. For example, a subcommittee to address ventilator-associated pneumonia may be formed from the Patient Safety Committee. This new group would be charged with a specific task that falls under the goals and purpose of the larger group. Once the ad hoc committee has addressed the topic, the ad hoc group would disband. In this example, responsibility for ongoing monitoring of improved outcomes related to ventilator-associated pneumonia would return to the larger Patient Safety Committee.

CNSs also lead groups that do not consist of meetings and agendas, such as a multidisciplinary rounding team. In this situation many of the same principles of groups apply. A multidisciplinary rounding team still needs clear vision and purpose, defined membership, a predetermined schedule, and, above all, leadership.

Chartering Your Group

A charter is a way to organize a group so that the key elements are well defined and communicated. Start by asking, "What is the *purpose* of this group?" It is very important that the group you are leading be thoughtfully constructed and have clear direction. The group must also fit with the goals, vision, and mission of the organization, committee, or unit that it is intended to serve. The group's purpose may be delegated by an administrator or written into organizational bylaws. However, for situations in which a CNS identifies a need to develop a group to fill a distinct need, the purpose should be developed by its members within the group. Regardless of the reason for the group, it is essential that those who elect or are appointed to participate in the group know, understand, and agree upon the purpose of the group and the end product or *deliverables* expected.

Who should be the *members* of the group? CNSs bring leadership and clinical talent to a group; however, CNSs do not work in isolation. Collaboration and teamwork are essential to achieving high-quality outcomes and cost control in client care (Huber, 2000). A diverse group of professionals collectively possesses greater knowledge and information, increases the likelihood of acceptance and understanding of the decisions made by the group, and enhances cooperation in implementation of any plan or intervention (Sullivan & Decker, 2005).

When deciding who should be in the group, first determine any standing members or required members. For some committees, bylaws or accreditation guidelines may specify members—not the individual person, but the credentials of the person. For example, accreditation guidelines may specify that some committees include physician members, while other committees may specify interdisciplinary membership. In addition to determining the required members, assess the stakeholders associated with the group's purpose and expected outcome. Make sure all key stakeholders have a voice in the group. It is easy to have too many members in a group—groups between 4 and 12 individuals are the most efficient; however, some groups necessitate a much larger population of members and can work very well (Marrelli, 2004). Giving voice to all stakeholders without adding members requires some thoughtful consideration. It may be necessary to select only one person from a large stakeholder group and charge this person with communicating with key members of the larger group, or the group may decide to publish reports, hold informational meetings, or seek input and feedback from stakeholders in other ways. In the end, a CNS should help ensure that the group is not overpopulated, does not include unnecessary members, and is not missing important key stakeholders.

Avoid the temptation to rely on established clinical leaders or administrators to participate in the group. As much as these members add strength to the group, it is essential that you include the "end users"—those persons who work with the targeted patient population and will be responsible for implementing the outcomes of the group's work. For example, when organizing a group to plan for medication reconciliation, those clinicians who will implement the plan developed by the group should be included. Including direct caregivers may create some challenges in scheduling meetings; however, caregivers can provide vital information that helps shape the work of the team and leads to better acceptance during the implementation phase. Clearly communicating the group members' expectations, including time commitments, may help avoid poor attendance and/or lack of participation. Change the day or time that the group meets, if necessary, to motivate individuals who may be reluctant due to scheduling concerns. Give members clear assignments with timelines and benchmarks for accountability. CNSs are group leaders and should keep the group goals moving forward; avoid or promptly resolve individual issues that create obstacles in meeting goals and timelines.

At times, a CNS may need to invite ad hoc members to join the group for a short period of time. For example, when reviewing data to determine responses to emergency situations, if the group identifies telecommunications issues that are slowing response times, the group should ask a member of the telecommunications department to join the group to brainstorm and problem solve these specific issues. Once the issues are resolved, the ad hoc member may be excused. It is important to be respectful of everyone's time. It may be necessary for selected key individuals to be present for only part of a meeting, during which a particular agenda's items are addressed, or it may not be necessary for some members to attend every meeting. Let the agenda guide the attendance for each meeting.

Schedules need to be determined well ahead of time. The frequency of meeting should be determined by the nature and urgency of the work. For example, a multidisciplinary rounding team may need to assemble twice a week in order to accomplish patient care plan revisions, whereas a departmental committee with the primary purpose of approving policies may have to meet only every other month. The time of day at which your group meets should be carefully considered. Groups that have physician members tend to be better attended early in the morning. Scheduling meetings for groups that contain members that work various shifts can be challenging. Work with the unit manager to plan appropriately to allow for staff nurses to participate in group work.

The *agenda* of any meeting should be driven by the purpose for which the group was formed. Agendas should be distributed before the meeting (usually 1 week) in order to give members time to prepare and thoughtfully consider the items. Depending on the group's charter, members may be able to contribute to or amend the agenda. Items should be prioritized on the agenda to allow enough time to address all items on the list. Standing reports and recurring updates can be distributed with the agenda as written reports, thus maximizing group interactions during the meeting. For each item, indicate the time allotted and the person responsible for presenting or reporting on that topic. To relay the purpose of each agenda item, use decisive phrases such as "to recommend" or "to make a final decision" for those items in which action is expected, and "to discuss" or "to consider" for those in which the purpose is *not* to drive action (McConnell, 2006). In this way, the group members are given a clear message about what the expected outcome is for the topics included in the meeting.

Discussion and Follow-Up

The scope, function, and authority of the group must be clearly stated (Liebler & McConnell, 2004). Is the purpose of the group to deliberate and make recommendations; does it have the authority to make decisions that are binding? If the purpose is to formulate recommendations, it must be clear to whom those recommendations are to be given. To whom is the group accountable? As the group leader, you are responsible for communicating the vision, strategy, and outcomes of your team to the person or group to whom the group is accountable.

Whatever group a CNS is leading, there must be a clear understanding of the group's decision-making authority. The group's authority will depend on the status of the members of the group, the nature of the decisions, and the impact of those decisions on the organization. If the group is not able to implement decisions, a CNS may need to secure an administrative sponsor. If the group's work involves expectations from physician colleagues, securing a physician champion is a wise move as well.

Groups may have a very formal process structure, or it may be very informal. As with membership, the structure of the group may be determined by bylaws or accreditation guidelines or other influences. The final structure depends on the authority and charge of the group. For instance, a board of directors that has administrative and fiscal responsibility for an organization is a very structured group. There are required agenda items, and minutes must be taken, approved, and archived. Standing committees usually require minutes that include attendance, discussion topics, and decisions or actions that result from committee voting. Task groups and ad hoc groups may not need minutes; these groups may submit one final report to the primary committee or administrator.

Documentation

It is good practice to document the work of every group. When minutes are required, it is very difficult for one person to both facilitate a meeting and take minutes, so a CNS should secure clerical support whenever possible. If this cannot be accomplished, ask for a volunteer from the group to take minutes. Keep in mind that the documentation of the proceedings may serve as the evidence that accreditation standards are being met. Therefore, minutes should be accurate, specific, detailed, and reflect all decisions and action plans with responsible persons assigned to them. Some key elements that should be contained in the minutes are as follows:

- Name of the group
- Date and location of the meeting
- Time the meeting started and adjourned
- Attendance: list those present as well as those who were absent (be sure to note absences as excused or not excused)
- Any guests or substitute members in attendance
- A statement that the previous minutes were approved
- Discussion topics and discussion leader
- A summary of the discussion and any subsequent decisions made—be sure to document the final decision that was made
- All actions to be taken, with responsible party and time frame in which the action should be completed
- Items to be continued onto the next meeting's agenda
- Date, place, and time of the next meeting

Minutes should be made available to members within a reasonable time frame and retained in accordance with your organization's document retention policy (usually between 3 and 5 years).

Environment and Setup

Ensure that the physical environment supports good group interaction. Make sure the temperature is acceptable and noise is kept to a minimum. Arranging seating in such a way that all members of the group can see one another often helps facilitate discussion and a feeling of equality among members. Classroom-type arrangements can suggest a lecturing environment, where one person dominates the discussion.

Because participants of meetings often work in multiple different buildings or off-site locations, gathering members in one location can present challenges. Although it is not ideal, consider substituting some face-to-face meetings for conference calls or allow some members from more distant sites to join by telephone. Consider the impact it may have on the group dynamics or meeting agenda before proceeding. Keep in mind that meetings that include brainstorming or flowcharting processes are difficult to conduct using phone conference methods. When using phone conferencing technology, be sure to send any documents to the member(s) before the meeting.

Securing Resources

The formation of a work group is not without cost to the organization. Therefore, a group must be efficient in accomplishing its goals and meeting the overall purpose. As the leader, you are responsible for articulating the value and impact that a group has on your organization and obtaining the resources necessary to efficiently accomplish the work of the group. One important resource is clerical support to help with the operational elements of the group work. In addition to writing minutes, a clerical assistant can arrange for meeting space, prepare materials, and assist with communications with others.

Good group meetings can be enhanced by ensuring that the appropriate equipment and supplies are available. Easels and flip charts can be essential in documenting brainstorming sessions. Electronic equipment such as computers and LCD panels can enhance the effectiveness of group presentations. Plan ahead and have all necessary equipment and supplies available. Test electronic equipment prior to the meeting to avoid wasting time troubleshooting mechanical failures or replacing missing items.

Leader Responsibilities

The leader sets the tone of the meeting. Start and end meetings promptly. Starting late gives positive reinforcement to latecomers. Establish a clear expectation that meetings will start on time, and members will quickly adjust their schedules to avoid being late. Most meetings typically last between 60 and 90 minutes. If the meeting is to exceed 90 minutes, time for a break should be allotted in the schedule.

Open meetings by concisely and clearly communicating an overview of the focus, task, or agenda for the meeting. During a meeting, summarize decisions and action items to bring clarity to discussions, to reinforce individual responsibility for action items, and to assist in accurately recording minutes. At the end of the meeting, read out loud a list of action items and the person responsible for each item.

Setting the milieu is also the responsibility of the group leader. Simple gestures such as thanking members for their attendance and recognizing individuals for their effort and contribution will facilitate a feeling of worth and appreciation among members. Expressions of appreciation will encourage quality performance and set a precedent for how all group members should interact with one another.

Soliciting ideas, opinions, and information prior to a meeting can be helpful. For example, if a CNS is facilitating a health care agency's emergency response committee and the agenda includes approving a new outline for advanced cardiac life support classes, it may be valuable to send the proposed course outline to members of the committee for feedback prior to the meeting. Sending an advance copy for review should facilitate more thoughtful discussion; provide opportunity for members to validate concerns by checking existing guidelines, empiric evidence, or expert opinion; and thus make for more considered discussion at the meeting.

Some other responsibilities of the group leader are:

- Periodically review team progress and goal attainment
- Respond enthusiastically to all suggestions and ideas of group members
- Allow everyone in the group the opportunity to be heard
- Entertain various problem-solving methods and potential solutions
- Do not give your opinion until everyone else has spoken
- Keep track of the time and keep on schedule
- Assign tasks as needed
- Role model and inspire others to continue their focus on the goals of the group
- Correlate group activities with the work of other related groups or departments
- Ensure compliance with mandated expectations and deadlines

Remember, groups that are productive tend to build on ideas of members by finding the strengths in a suggestion. In groups that are not productive, members spend time finding the weaknesses of an idea. A CNS can facilitate a productive group by asking members to build on ideas with statements like "What is good about that idea" or "How can we strengthen that idea so it will work with our patients." Keep the creative juices flowing by rewarding innovative thinking and minimizing devil's advocate-type arguments.

Group Member Responsibilities

For staff nurses and others, being selected to serve as a group member should be viewed as an honor. Members possess the important knowledge and skills needed for a specific outcome. As group leaders, CNSs should communicate that being a member of a group is important and comes with responsibilities. Make sure the members of the group know the expectations and responsibilities of membership.

Attendance at group meetings is a clear expectation. Some absences are expected; however, members should send a designated representative to a meeting when appropriate. In some situations, for attendance purposes a member who sends a designated representative may be considered an excused absence (in lieu of unexcused absence). Continued membership on a committee or work group may be dependent on attendance; after a specified number of unexcused absences (often 3), the member is removed from the committee. The attendance requirement and consequences should be stated up front.

Group members should come to meetings prepared to participate. This means having obtained and/or read all pertinent materials ahead of time. For example, if a policy is to be approved during a meeting, time to read the policy will not be available during the meeting—the meeting will include discussion and voting on action items only. Members should also prepare by obtaining additional information to answer any questions, validate concerns, or identify alternatives. Being prepared to offer ideas that address problem areas will keep the work of the committee moving forward.

Group members should actively participate in discussions by offering feedback, suggestions, and ideas in a respectful and professional manner. This may be difficult for members new to communicating ideas in groups. When a committee includes inexperienced members, a CNS leader should be creative in assisting these members to contribute. Actively seeking ideas by calling upon individuals or using a *round robin* approach to solicit input from the less verbal members of the group may be helpful in drawing out new members. It is equally important to control the talkers in the group so everyone has a chance to contribute.

Although the group leader is responsible for keeping meetings on track, it is also the responsibility of each group member to help the discussion stay on topic and to the point. It is not helpful for any member of the group (including the leader) to get sidetracked by tangents or "soap box" lectures. As the leader, avoid these non-constructive behaviors and stop others by bringing them back to the initial topic. Some tangential conversations may actually be good agenda items for future meetings, so consider suggesting adding the topic to a future agenda.

As the leader, clearly communicate the expectation that members complete assigned action items/tasks. Group progress slows when assignments are not completed in a timely manner. If group members repeatedly fail to complete assignments, the leader must intervene. Confront member(s) in a private setting using a non-threatening and caring manner. Give the member the opportunity to explain why the task was not completed. It could be that the member did not understand the task, did not have adequate resources, or was faced with unplanned or uncontrollable circumstances that prevented the work from being finished. Give the member an opportunity to reflect on why the task was not completed and to either renew his/her commitment to complete the task or hand it off with no repercussions. If the member demonstrates a pattern of completing work late or failing to complete work, the CNS should suggest that this may not be the best time for the person to serve on the committee/group. Resignation will facilitate appointment of a new member until such time as the person can devote more time and energy to the group.

Finally, where the group is charged with implementation, members should understand that it is an expectation that they assist with implementation of action plans. Members should become champions of the change and resources for implementation within their peer groups. Members should seek feedback about both the implementation process and the action plan itself. The group should also facilitate collecting and analyzing evaluation data and reporting.

Mentoring New Group Leaders

Members of the group should be given opportunities to develop professionally, and CNSs can make good mentors. As you gain experience as a CNS group leader, try giving some members assignments that you typically would perform. For example, ask one or two group members to conduct a literature review or search for guidelines or standards. Facilitate members in developing skills. Teaching staff nurses to perform literature reviews may take more of your time initially but is well worth the investment. Another way to mentor the group members and build skills is to rotate meeting leaders. Rotating leaders will give members opportunity to develop skills in conducting a meeting. As you identify the various strengths of the members, begin matching strengths with opportunities. For example, a member skilled at leading meetings could be asked to coordinate an ad hoc group to address a specific problem.

Revisiting Your Charter

Groups should be subject to periodic review of purpose and function (Liebler & McConnell, 2004). This review may help to either acknowledge the importance of the group or provide redirection. In evaluating the group, ask:

- Do the proceedings and production of the group still fit with the purpose, goals, and mission that were originally outlined?
- Would the organization be affected if this group were eliminated?
- Do meeting frequency, day, and time meet with the needs of the members and organization?
- Is the group the right size and are the necessary stakeholders present?

If the answer to any of these questions is no, you may want to consider changes. Present the analysis to the group for discussion, and share findings with the person to whom the group is accountable.

I hope that you have enjoyed this summary on leading groups. The CNS is ideal for this role and can make an impact on an organization as both a formal and informal leader. It has been my pleasure to work with some phenomenal groups in some fantastic work in my organization. Good luck in all your endeavors!

References

Huber, D. (2000). *Leadership and nursing care management* (2nd ed.). Philadelphia: W. B. Saunders Company.

Liebler, J. G., & McConnell, C. R. (2004). *Management principles for health professionals* (4th ed.). Boston: Jones and Bartlett.

Marrelli, T. M. (2004). *The nurse manager's survival guide: Practical answers to everyday problems* (3rd ed.). St. Louis: Mosby.

McConnell, C. R. (2006). *Umiker's management skills for the new health care supervisor* (4th ed.). Boston: Jones and Bartlett.

National Association of Clinical Nurse Specialists (NACNS). (2004). *Statement on clinical nurse specialist practice and education* (2nd ed.). Harrisburg, PA: Author.

Sullivan, E. J., & Decker, P. J. (2005). *Effective leadership and management in nursing* (6th ed.). Upper Saddle River, NJ: Pearson Education.

11

Mentoring Staff

Patricia A. Foster

Clinical nurse specialists (CNSs) know something important about staff success with patient care—the power of mentoring. Consider this mentoring experience: Peggy, an experienced registered nurse (RN), started orientation as a staff nurse in a hemodialysis unit. During Peggy's clinical orientation, she had two CNS mentors: Diane and Nancy. Diane was patient, explained the steps of dialysis treatments, and provided encouragement as Peggy learned to use the equipment. On the other hand, Nancy sternly questioned Peggy about each step during the dialysis treatment and never provided any encouragement to her. For example, Nancy always questioned Peggy about the patient's post-dialysis weight by saying, "Are you sure that is correct? That doesn't sound right to me." Often as Peggy left work, she was in tears wondering if she "had what it takes" to work as a dialysis nurse in this unit. Based on this mentoring experience, how would you, as a CNS, mentor Peggy so she would not become discouraged to the point of leaving dialysis nursing? Being a mentor to staff can help them succeed in their work environment.

Katz (2001) describes mentoring as a personal as well as professional relationship characterized by mutual respect, trust, understanding, and empathy. An effective mentor is respected, reliable, patient, trustworthy, and a very good listener and communicator. CNSs, with their clinical expertise, are among the best mentors in a clinical setting. We understand that our interactions with staff are opportunities to help them discover their potential at work and in their professional career.

As a CNS, you have the opportunity, by mentoring staff, to directly affect the quality of care for that patient while simultaneously supporting patient safety. This chapter describes: (a) how you can develop a "mentoring perspective," (b) what the essential qualities for being a mentor are, (c) what to consider when developing a mentoring plan, (d) myths about mentoring, (e) "mentoring on the move" strategies, and (f) how to know if you are already mentoring staff but have not realized it.

Developing a Mentoring Perspective

As CNSs, we work in a variety of different settings, clinical areas, and specialties. While we differ in our kind of work, we all share a responsibility and commitment to serve as mentors to staff. Whereas health care has undergone various changes throughout the years, one CNS responsibility that has remained constant is the mentoring of staff. Mentoring is essential for staff nurses to succeed in the development of their professional career. One of your most important roles as a CNS is to serve as a mentor for staff. Not only do you serve as a role model to exemplify what it means to be a successful nurse, but also you serve as a potential ally and advocate for all staff that you encounter.

Does mentoring mean you will have to do mentoring duties in addition to your other responsibilities that you already have? No, not at all. Mentoring is not a separate set of activities, but rather it involves how you think and feel about staff and yourself. Most important, mentoring deals with how you, as a CNS, communicate with staff.

In addition, mentoring does not mean that you will have to spend huge amounts of time with individual staff, nor does it mean that you will have to mentor all new staff that you meet. What mentoring does mean is that you make every effort to ensure that each contact you make with staff counts. It is not the quantity, but the quality of time you spend with staff that sets mentoring apart from other kinds of activities. In other words, every time you meet a nurse there is a potential opportunity for mentoring. The mentoring process does not require separate meetings where you purposely act as a role model. Whatever setting or reason you have to talk with a nurse, through your words and actions you will have the opportunity to serve as a mentor. Mentoring is a reciprocal relationship where both the CNS and staff benefit and learn from one another. As a CNS, you have the opportunity to make a difference in the lives of staff by serving as a mentor.

Essential Qualities for Being a Mentor

According to Butler and Felts (2006), essential qualities of a mentor include: (a) nurturing the staff, (b) acting as a close, trusted, and experienced clinical guide, (c) encouraging, teaching, and leading staff through significant points in their careers, (d) teaching by example, (e) acting as a sounding board, (f) giving honest feedback, and (g) helping the staff establish themselves in their profession. How do CNSs apply these mentoring qualities in the workplace?

Nurturing the staff is how CNSs provide support to staff in the clinical setting. Remember how it felt when you were in orientation and a helpful mentor taught you how to start the intravenous saline lock? In addition, the mentor was encouraging, taught you about the "unwritten rules" of the unit, introduced you to other staff, and made you feel part of the team. Nurturing is providing a safe haven in which staff know they are safe and understand it is okay to ask questions. CNSs practice unconditional acceptance of the nurses as people while providing expert guidance on the necessary skills to work in a clinical area.

The second quality of acting as a close, trusted, and experienced guide speaks to the essential role of the CNS—the clinical expertise. Here is where your experience of doing a procedure "many times" really shines. The CNS can tell novice staff about those tips to make a procedure seem effortless. For example, a novice RN inserting a nasogastric (N/G) tube but not getting a fluid return after it is connected to wall suction will call the CNS. Upon arriving at the patient's bedside, the CNS observes an anxious RN. The CNS performs a quick assessment of the problem and finds the N/G tube coiled in the patient's throat and removes it. Next, in a private setting, the CNS determines the RN's skills with N/G tube insertion. The new RN says, "I placed one N/G tube as a nursing student but that was over three years ago." The CNS determines the new RN does not have sufficient knowledge and skills to insert an N/G tube, so she performs the procedure while creating a teaching moment for the new RN. The CNS provides time afterward to answer any questions the new RN may have. Two days later, the new RN pages the CNS about another N/G insertion she needs to do. The CNS and the new RN review a plan to support the new RN during the procedure. The plan involves the CNS standing across the bed from the new RN and explaining to the patient, step by step, what will happen during the N/G insertion procedure. The procedure steps are reviewed before entering the patient's room. While the RN sets up the equipment, the CNS talks with the patient by saying, "Hi, my name is Janet and I am a clinical nurse specialist who will be assisting Mary, your nurse, as she places the N/G tube. What I want you to do is to listen to me as I tell you what is happening so you will know when to take a sip of water and hold your breath. Is this okay with you?" The patient says yes. Janet, the CNS, has the patient's attention and cooperation as the nurse inserts the N/G tube. The new nurse listens to what Janet is telling the patient about what will happen next—a form of real-time coaching. Once the N/G insertion procedure is completed, the CNS and the RN meet briefly to evaluate the insertion procedure. In this scenario, the CNS demonstrates clinical expertise while mentoring staff competency and patient safety to create a win-win situation.

A third quality is the CNS helping guide staff through important phases of their professional career. Key points for the CNS: Provide an opportunity for staff to talk with you; listen to problems; identify what needs to be done and provide resources. An example would be a graduate nurse who has taken the NCLEX licensing examination but did not receive a passing score. The CNS explores with the graduate nurse what factors may have contributed to the low NCLEX score and discovers that the graduate nurse becomes extremely anxious during examinations, especially when they are timed tests. The CNS could suggest a

NCLEX refresher class along with handouts or books on test-taking strategies to reduce testing stress and anxiety.

Teaching by example, the fourth quality, is an area where CNSs excel. CNSs have been teaching since they first started out on a nursing career. Almost daily, we teach patients about the medications they are taking, families how to change a dressing, and other staff as we learn about new equipment. In addition, your CNS program provided you with knowledge about patient teaching that you used in your clinicals. You have been teaching your entire nursing career.

The fifth quality, acting as a "sounding board," is an important quality for a CNS to use in the clinical setting. By understanding the clinical issues you can help prepare the staff to succeed in their work environment. For example, join staff in the break room and listen to what they are talking about and learn about their issues.

Giving honest feedback creates a trusting relationship with staff. Nurses want to know about changes in their practice that affect quality care and patient safety. When staff discuss a clinical problem, consider sharing examples of "I might do this" scenarios to help staff learn about different ways to deal with the problem.

Finally, CNSs serve as role models for staff when it comes to establishing themselves in their profession. Help staff to find information about certification in a clinical specialty. If you are certified, share your experiences regarding how you prepared for your certification testing. Encourage staff to join professional nursing organizations and help them find information about them.

Developing a Mentoring Plan

When mentoring staff, CNSs should develop a plan with objectives. Here are four objectives to consider as you create your plan:

1. Establish a positive personal relationship with all staff you meet.

    ■ Avoid acting as if you are nothing more than a professional service provider ("I'm here to do a job. I'm not here to be your friend!"). Make a proactive effort to act as a guide, a coach, an ally, and an advocate.
    ■ Trust and respect must be established. Be aware it takes time for staff to get to know you and how a CNS can help them. Take every opportunity to teach staff about the CNS role and what you can do for them.
    ■ Regular interaction and consistent support are important in mentoring relationships. As you round in departments, take time to stop and listen to staff tell you about what is happening in their area.
    ■ Once you have developed a positive personal relationship, it is much easier to realize the remaining three goals.

2. Help staff develop career and life skills.

    ■ Work to accomplish specific goals for staff (i.e., staff understanding how to manage chest tube drainage systems).

- When appropriate, emphasize critical thinking skills such as decision making, goal setting, time management, dealing with conflict, and skills for coping with stress and fear (i.e., give them examples of how you managed your time as a staff nurse by sharing a story they can relate to).

3. Assist staff in locating clinical and hospital resources.

- Provide information or help your staff find clinical resources (doctors, staff, policies and procedures, support services, professional organizations, etc.). Next, assist your staff in learning how to access and use these resources (i.e., sit down at a computer and show them how to locate the online policy for blood transfusion or how to register for an online class).

4. Enhance your staff's ability to interact comfortably and productively with people from diverse racial, ethnic, cultural, and socioeconomic backgrounds.

- Your willingness as a CNS to interact with people different from yourself will make a powerful statement about the values placed on diversity. Role model the attitudes and behaviors that you emphasize (i.e., during rounds make time to talk with international nurses as well as new nurse graduates).
- Acknowledge and understand, not ignore, our cultural differences. Learn how to use our differences as resources for growth to produce new understandings and insights. An international nurse told me, "It seems so lonely in American hospitals because all patients do not have family with them at all times." Her comment reminded me to take time to talk with those patients who have no visitors.
- Everyone holds preconceptions and stereotypes about one's own group and other groups. Take special care that you, as a CNS, are not (intentionally or unintentionally) promoting your views at the expense of your staff's viewpoints. Work on understanding and critically examining your own perspectives on race, ethnicity, culture, class, religion, sexual orientation, etc.

Mentoring Misconceptions

When one thinks of a mentor, it conjures up certain unfounded beliefs about who is a mentor and what qualities a mentor possesses. Here are some mentoring myths:

Misconception: In a hospital, you need to be an older person with gray hair (or no hair) to be a good mentor.
Reality: In a hospital, mentors can be young or old. Some of the most outstanding mentors are your CNS colleagues, regardless of age.
Misconception: Mentoring only happens one-to-one on a long-term basis.
Reality: In a hospital, mentoring occurs in many different ways. Some mentoring relationships are traditional relationships involving a one-to-one

relationship over a long period. However, effective mentoring can also occur in a group setting or even through a single encounter with a nurse. As a CNS, use each encounter with staff as an opportunity for mentoring and think about ways to infuse mentoring into your daily work.

Misconception: Only the person being mentored benefits from mentoring.

Reality: By definition, mentoring is a reciprocal relationship where both the CNS mentor and the nurse learn from each other. True mentors are those who have developed the wisdom to learn from those they mentor.

Misconception: CNSs already have many responsibilities related to staff education and do not have the time to take on extra responsibilities related to mentoring.

Reality: Mentoring is not a separate set of activities that are different from other job responsibilities. Mentoring relates to the consciousness about one's work as a CNS and being a trusted ally to staff. Without this consciousness, staff see CNSs as bureaucrats focusing on rules, regulations, and procedures. Hospitals do not need more bureaucrats. Hospitals do need CNSs who are staff-centered and who can see and nurture the potential in others.

Misconception: By calling yourself a mentor, you become a mentor.

Reality: Not all CNSs who work with staff are mentors, even if they have that job title. Mentors are those who have developed consciousness about mentoring and in their interactions with staff demonstrate respect, patience, trustworthiness, and strong communication skills, especially listening skills.

Misconception: To become a mentor requires a lot of time and work.

Reality: Becoming a mentor requires a change in consciousness, that is, how you think about yourself and how you think about others. Mentoring is not a matter of working harder or longer or adding to your job responsibilities but seeing your work differently.

Misconception: At a large hospital, one CNS can mentor only a limited number of staff. Although a CNS may want to help large numbers of staff, the cold reality is that she or he can only work with a select few.

Reality: Every single encounter with a staff member is a mentoring opportunity. The key is to develop consciousness about the importance of mentoring during your interactions with staff and to infuse this consciousness into your daily work as a CNS. In addition, it is important for CNSs to see themselves as part of a CNS network—as part of a community of mentors. To effectively help a particular nurse, a CNS mentor can draw upon this network or community. Mentoring occurs in a community, not in isolation.

Mentoring on the Move

Mentoring on the move describes ways a CNS can effectively mentor staff anywhere their work takes them that day. Here are some strategies to consider when you are mentoring on the move in your hospital:

- Include mentoring in everyday staff interactions (i.e., rounding, at the nurse's station, and helping with procedures).

- Mentoring occurs every day, in many forms and ways. Mentoring can take place in a brief encounter that may have a powerful impact on the nurse you mentor.
- Mentoring works most effectively when it is done with purpose (i.e., teaching a new skill, collaborating on an evidence-based project, demonstrating use of new equipment, pursuing a common interest). Just as often, mentoring without a specific purpose can work (i.e., being available as a "sounding board").
- Issues related to diversity are key for CNSs. Sometimes diversity is viewed as a problem rather than an opportunity for enriching teaching and mentoring. For example, in a Preceptor Class, I used a discussion panel of nurses who were experienced preceptors, new graduate nurses, and international nurses.
- The timing of mentoring can be crucial. Mentoring may need to follow when staff learn how to use new equipment or a new protocol (i.e., changing from paper to electronic charting requires frequent "on the spot" mentoring).
- Nurses who need the most mentoring are precisely those who "fall between the cracks" (i.e., staff who have not been trained on new equipment or a new protocol).

You Are Mentoring Staff When ...

Every day CNSs interact with staff, patients, families, physicians, and other health care workers throughout the hospital. Every time a CNS makes contact with another person, there is a potential mentoring moment, but the CNS may not recognize it. You are mentoring staff when ...

- You help staff achieve potential within themselves that is hidden to others—and perhaps themselves.
- You share stories with staff about your own career and the ways you overcame obstacles that are similar to the ones they are encountering.
- You help staff overcome their fear of a coworker and help them to learn ways to deal with difficult personalities.
- You show staff how you learned time management when you worked as a staff nurse.
- You listen to a staff nurse describe a clinical problem and then explore resources at the hospital to help the staff nurse deal with the problem.
- You help a new staff nurse understand a particularly tough procedure— and explain it in such a way that the nurse is willing to come back to you when there is another difficult skill to learn.
- You know more about the staff nurse's clinical skills than what the nurse tells you.

Summary

CNSs advance nursing practice, improve clinical outcomes, and provide clinical expertise to staff on a daily basis. Mentors should be good listeners, approachable by nursing staff, committed to the nursing profession, and team players as well as role models for expert clinical practice (Modic & Schloesser, 2007). By incorporating the strategies in this chapter into your practice, you will see the positive impact that mentoring staff will have in your organization.

References

Butler, M. R., & Felts, J. (2006). Tool kit for the staff mentor: Strategies for improving retention. *The Journal of Continuing Education, 37*(5), 210–213.

Katz, S. (2001). Acceptance: A mentor's joy and responsibilities. *Pediatric Research, 49*(5), 725–777.

Modic, M. B., & Schloesser, M. (2007). Preceptorship. *Journal for Staff Development, 23*(4), 195–196.

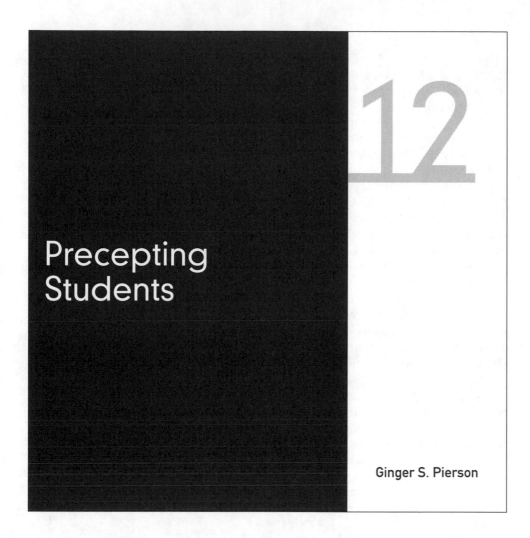

12

Precepting Students

Ginger S. Pierson

Knowledge and skills needed to practice as a clinical nurse specialist (CNS) effectively continue to expand as medical, nursing science, and technological innovations seem to be almost continual. Additionally, nursing now offers multiple creative educational entry tracts into the nursing profession, which may create unique challenges and opportunities. CNSs must have the ability to both mentor and precept clinical staff and graduate students seeking advanced practice as CNSs. Nurses in both education and clinical practice must create workplace environments that support professional nursing practice. An important hallmark of professional practice is creating a nurse-to-nurse mentoring environment, where experienced nurses are encouraged to share their knowledge, skills, and enthusiasm about professional nursing practice with nurses who are less experienced (American Association of Colleges of Nursing, 2002). Mentoring and precepting activities serve to promote a continual climate of excellence and a culture of encouragement, acceptance, and support for building new skills (Firtko, Stewart, & Knox, 2005). Myrick and Yonge (2004) emphasize that "the relationship that evolved during the preceptorship experience was found to be pivotal not only to the enhancement of critical thinking, but also to the success of the experience and the student's own sense of professional competence"

(p. 374). CNSs should embrace and practice critical thinking to foster growth in CNS graduate students as they learn the CNS advanced practice role and responsibilities.

Clinical currency and great flexibility/adaptability in CNS practice are highly valued and expected in your role and specialty. Clinical expertise within a specialty enables CNSs to provide expert advanced care to patients and clients to positively affect the delivery of care and resultant outcomes. These are often based on standards of care developed from best evidence-based practices (National Association of Clinical Nurse Specialists [NACNS], 2004). CNS skills are attained through extensive clinical experience as a bedside RN and then further developed as a CNS, with ongoing review of the literature for the latest evidence-based practices, networking with CNS colleagues, and active involvement in professional nursing organizations. These reflect some of the core components for effective CNS role development and implementation into practice. It is crucial to impart a foundation of these elements to CNS graduate students during their clinical preceptorship with advanced practice nurses, as CNSs implement their unique practice in very different ways and settings. Serving as a preceptor for graduate CNS students is a great honor and a professional responsibility. It carries with it accountability for thorough exposure to the role of the CNS. Time must be planned to show how the CNS role contributes to or impacts each of the three key spheres of influence: the patient/client sphere, the nurses/nursing sphere, and the system/organizational sphere (NACNS, 2004). Advance planning and ongoing discussion before and during the clinical rotation help define clear goals and direction for an effective CNS preceptor and CNS graduate student partnership. Five phases to serve as a guide for this partnership will be discussed: becoming a CNS preceptor, defining the CNS/graduate student relationship and setting goals, active participation in the CNS role, professional association involvement, and evaluation of the clinical partnership experience.

Becoming a CNS Preceptor

The CNS may want to consider spending the first year as a CNS in practice without precepting a CNS graduate student. Time during this first year is needed for focused attention on adjusting to and refining the role/contributions within the organization as a CNS. This might be the first CNS role for the organization, or you may be replacing an experienced CNS with much history and expectation from the organization or units/patient populations served.

Once you are settled into the role of CNS, precepting a CNS graduate may then seem possible and desirable. Discuss this commitment with your chief nurse officer or other appropriate supervisor (to whomever you report). Gain support for your planned preceptor and graduate student partnership, and consider how it will affect your role regarding time, projects, and plans for CNS student involvement in all CNS activities and meetings. Involvement of other key nursing directors/leaders may also be necessary. This may include, for example, the director of nursing education, who may organize all nursing student academic contracts—including required school/hospital contract agreements, immunizations, background checks, confidentiality agreements, and more—prior to the student's start of the clinical rotation. Key aspects of hospital/nursing orientation, depending on the scope of the CNS practice/setting, may also be required for the CNS graduate student prior to start of clinical. Most hospital organizations will welcome the opportunity of hosting CNS graduate students—sharing in their clinical development and experience. This may also be an effective recruitment tool for future CNS positions for the organization.

Once organizational readiness has been obtained to host CNS graduate students at your hospital/facility, contact the program chair of CNS graduate schools in your area and discuss serving as a clinical preceptor for CNS graduate students. When the CNS clinical instructor contacts you, provide a detailed description of your experience as an RN, your experience as a CNS, and your current role responsibilities. This will provide the instructor with appropriate information to assign a CNS graduate student to best develop an effective clinical partnership. Preceptor agreements and copies of your curriculum vitae or resume are usually required for academic files.

Defining the CNS/Graduate Student Relationship and Setting Goals

The CNS preceptor and CNS student relationship requires effective communication skills, trust, flexibility, and some interpersonal risk. Mutual respect fosters creative thinking and allows for achievement of high expectations of the CNS role. The role of the CNS student is to accept responsibility for learning and to be actively engaged in the clinical experience with great interest and curiosity. The student should also have an ability to self-reflect on performance and accept and give feedback regarding the clinical experience (Butler & Felts, 2006).

Initial phone or e-mail contact is often established at least 1 to 2 months prior to the start of the clinical rotation. First priorities focus on completing required institutional contract requirements for the rotation and plans for any required hospital/nursing orientation. These should be discussed and dates for completion established. Further introductions are now necessary regarding each other's clinical experience as an RN and as a CNS/graduate student to find common ground to relate. The CNS student is always very interested to learn up front some details of your various functions and responsibilities as a CNS and how he or she may become involved. Care should be taken to not overwhelm the student with too much detail to start, but just introduce broad responsibilities and projects of interest based on the student's background and anticipated class objectives.

Often during this initial phone or e-mail contact, the CNS student has not started class yet and does not know details for the clinical rotation other than start and end dates, total number of clinical hours needed, and recommended number of clinical days per week to achieve the course goals. Specific objectives or projects that are required may not be known at this time. Initial dates for the first several clinical shifts are suggested at this time—based on the CNS's schedule/availability. This may allow for further planning for the student, who may also have a work schedule to consider in addition to graduate school, family, and other commitments.

On the first day of clinical with the CNS graduate student, an orientation plan should be created or reviewed for the clinical preceptorship, including plans for the evaluation process and the individual's learning style and preferences. A description of expectations for your CNS preceptor role and what is expected for the graduate student should be discussed and clarified. Dialogue throughout the clinical preceptorship should be ongoing between the CNS preceptor and the orientee. Feedback should be provided daily and progress discussed formally, often weekly or on a regular basis, throughout the preceptorship. Reassure the CNS graduate student that any mistakes are kept confidential but reviewed to examine alternative decisions, actions, and possible outcomes (Modic & Harris, 2007). Immediate feedback is most productive and useful when reviewed just after the situation has occurred. This allows reflective thoughts at a time when recall is still fresh, honest, accurate, and relevant, to correct and positively affect current knowledge and future clinical experiences (Brown, 2007).

Time should be planned in the first 1 or 2 days together to review academic course objectives and required projects, as well as any further mutual expectations. One to two hours minimum is commonly needed to start this process. Further specific expectations to be discussed may include clinical hours to be spent and possible flexibility as desired (more concentrated clinical for most weeks or spread out evenly over entire rotation), a communication plan for absence/late for clinical, plan for best communication method between planned clinical shifts, professional behavior, confidentiality, communication and attire during clinical rotation, and expected follow-through on independent and collaborative projects.

During this first or second meeting, the CNS student is often unsure of the expectations for the clinical course and tries to discover what the objectives/ projects mean in terms of clinical practice. Sharing initial ideas about key projects you as a CNS are involved in helps at this early stage. Focus on those identified needs of your unit, patient population served, or the organization. This may help shape ideas for a brainstorming session for a follow-up meeting on the next clinical shift together. Identifying key project(s) early into the clinical rotation is critical to give the CNS student time to get involved and complete, or greatly contribute to, a clinical project that is of mutual interest and will be clinically useful to both parties. If the right project is chosen, the CNS student should feel excited to be involved with the project and, hopefully, can feel proud when sharing this accomplishment or contribution with the CNS faculty and other graduate students. These projects can be the start of developing a CNS portfolio of professional accomplishments and can be showcased in the interview process with future potential CNS employers. Additionally, the CNS graduate student should be encouraged to submit these completed projects to local and national CNS professional conferences as either poster or oral presentations to share ideas, strategies, and outcomes with other CNS colleagues. This creates early professional opportunities to present CNS accomplishments formally, facilitate networking with other CNSs, and spark interest and involvement in CNS organizations.

Active Participation in the CNS Role: Exposure to All Aspects of the Role

When a CNS graduate student comes to gain realistic clinical experience as a CNS, the student should be allowed to become involved in and exposed to as many aspects of the CNS role as possible. No meetings, activities, projects, or other involvement should be avoided because of possible sensitivities that may exist in the organization. Examples of these potentially sensitive situations may include MD or RN peer review sessions, counseling of employees with directors (i.e., establishing clinical learning contracts), multidisciplinary sentinel and clinical event meetings, and Joint Commission or Magnet survey processes or regulatory agency reviews. The CNS may need to discuss and obtain permission (usually from the chief nursing officer) to have the CNS student present at these meetings. Confidentiality agreements required for the organization may be signed by the CNS student at the start of the clinical rotation. This agreement should cover any sensitive confidentiality concerns. Further discussions regarding expectations or limitations in sharing information with fellow CNS students or faculty may also need to be addressed. Exposure to any or all of these situations allows the CNS student to observe and discuss the role and contributions in each situation with the CNS. These are great learning experiences not to be missed. Be proactive as the CNS preceptor and look for these and other unique learning opportunities. The CNS and the CNS graduate student should try to make an opportunity for a debriefing session following each meeting or regulatory survey. Discussion of overt/objective details covered in these meetings, as well as any subtle messages or interactions among team members, can provide valuable insight to the graduate student regarding group dynamics and navigating change in the organization.

Framework of Your CNS Role and Expectations

Providing a framework or overview of your CNS role, current projects, and activities early in the clinical experience can help the CNS student gain perspective of the CNS role in practice. This may be reviewed in a written format (ideal) or discussed verbally. Include how each role component may be organized as affecting each of NACNS's three spheres of influence (NACNS, 2004). An overview will help give the student an idea of the multiple roles and responsibilities the CNS is frequently involved with and will help the student focus on the current responsibilities/role component(s) encountered with each clinical day. Obtaining a copy of the CNS job description and/or annual evaluation tool for the CNS student may also help during this clinical rotation and future job interviews. Be sure to obtain permission from appropriate nurse leaders when sharing any organizational documents that may be considered sensitive or restricted by hospital/organizational policies. As clinical exposure of the CNS role grows, consider sharing how other CNSs in the organization, or other CNS professional colleagues, practice their roles differently: for example, unit-based CNSs, service-line-based CNSs, population-based CNSs, or other variation of CNS customer groups. Consider scheduling the graduate student with some clinical time (usually a half day or full day) with these other CNS colleagues, as available, to see their various activities, settings, and the customers they impact.

Planning Clinical Days Together

Flexibility of clinical days, when possible, may be best matched to known, planned CNS activities of interest for the CNS student, depending on availability for clinical. Graduate classes, work schedules, or family commitments may impact the schedule planned. Discuss availability or limitations to work night shifts, weekends, or other alternative hours. These may be regularly planned in the CNS schedule to provide CNS support to employees on all shifts as applicable to the CNS role. Scheduling several days together when time may be committed to focused clinical time on units/areas of responsibility is beneficial to prioritize. Additional time is also needed for discussion and work on clinical projects, for balancing ongoing time management of the CNS role, and for strategic planning. The CNS preceptor is expected to provide the daily clinical teaching with the graduate student but also has expectations from the unit/ organization to meet CNS clinical practice expectations for the role (Burns, Beauchesne, Ryan-Krause, & Sawin, 2006). Ongoing planning and flexibility by all help achieve these responsibilities.

Active Clinical Involvement, Visibility, and Maintaining Clinical Currency

The CNS is known for clinical expertise and clinical currency, which helps give great credibility in serving as a resource and role model for nurses in a specialty. Establishing this expertise and credibility is critical to the success of the CNS role in the organization. Graduate students must see and understand this vital component of the many CNS functions. Clinical competency and currency are often most highly valued by the CNS's direct customers: nurses, patients/ families, and the organization. Frequently working side-by-side with bedside nurses and sharing in all aspects of bedside care are especially important in the establishment of the perception/reality of CNS expertise, of the willingness to assist, and as a resource for all aspects of patient care related to the CNS's specialty area. This shared bedside care, involving the CNS and the staff nurse, allows the CNS to assess staff skills and develop a trusting and collaborative relationship. Maintaining clinical currency is reflected in assisted bedside practice in consultation roles, formal teaching of classes, informal teaching at the bedside, and in the identification and implementation of evidence-based clinical practice changes. Contributions involving the CNS's impact on clinical outcomes of patients and staff performance, on decreases in costs, and on patient length of stay are some of the many CNS role outcomes that may be measured to validate the direct CNS role contributions to the clinical areas of responsibility. The CNS must be actively involved in documenting leadership and participation in direct contributions to clinical excellence. Additionally, the CNS often provides leadership in applying evidence-based practice changes to clinical practice through formal organizational processes and use of change theory. Involvement of the CNS student in the planning and implementation of an evidence-based practice project during the clinical experience can greatly help the transition of knowledge (evidence-based practice theory) into clinical practice.

Further discussion of the frequent struggle to balance maximal clinical time on the units supporting staff and patients, to manage time preparing and teaching formal classes, to work on multiple projects, and to take care of committee responsibilities is important to share with the CNS student. Sharing time management strategies of the priorities most valued by the organization is crucial to the ongoing success of the CNS role and will be discussed further in this chapter.

Work on Committees and Projects

Involvement of the CNS student in ongoing committees may or may not be possible due to schedule conflicts, status of projects in process, or student preferences or interests. Much may be gained through attendance at committee meetings, such as use of CNS role in the committee; group dynamics, process, and politics; and evaluation of group leadership skills. These observations provide several possibilities for meaningful CNS dialogue for further role development of the CNS student.

CNS Education Role and Supportive Responsibilities

As previously mentioned, the CNS has an important role component in education—often in both formal teaching in the classroom and informal teaching done at the bedside with nurses and with patients and families. Some organizations/hospitals have nurse educators in separate supportive roles in addition to CNSs for specialty areas. An understanding of these separate, yet complementary roles, and their differences or the addition of all education responsibilities to the CNS role, is an important discussion to have with the CNS graduate student. This helps the student understand role responsibilities for maintaining required education records, documentation of completed orientation and required initial clinical competencies, annual competency skills or knowledge validation for Joint Commission or state regulatory agencies, and possible legal implications for the hospital in the future. When formal educator responsibilities are blended into the CNS role, reporting to a second director/manager for these education responsibilities may also occur. Discussion of ongoing reporting responsibilities and expected communication, as well as issues of overtime compensation (if applicable) by department and assessment of annual/ongoing performance evaluation, may assist the CNS student to explore and define expectations for future CNS interviews or job opportunities.

Prioritization of CNS Responsibilities and Time Management Strategies

A CNS student quickly learns during the clinical rotation that the CNS role is one of constant prioritization, time management, and required flexibility. As the CNS role is fully implemented and respected at the organization, multiple requests to involve the CNS's clinical expertise typically occur. Though viewed as a compliment to successful CNS role implementation and respect as a clinical expert, this can lead a CNS to be involved with too many educational classes or conferences, projects, committees, or other requests. This may also cause the CNS to lose focus of highest priority CNS responsibilities, as too many tasks and requests are trying to be achieved simultaneously. One strategy that has proved effective for some CNSs has been to visibly post hospital/organizational/unit goals and strategic vision in the office. A regular evaluation of each CNS activity can be listed and compared with these strategic goals/vision to distinguish whether the activity supports this planned direction. Those activities that do not support the strategic goals/vision should be reevaluated and discussed as to the CNS's continued involvement in the commitment. A proactive list of each CNS activity, committee, and project as they are added to the CNS's workload can be a supportive strategy for a new or overwhelmed CNS. This list may include headings such as Routine Tasks; Responsive (Time Limited) Tasks; Strategic Planning and Support for Goals/Vision (Campbell, 2006). Ongoing additions to this list may help provide the CNS with an immediate evaluation of the task/project in relation to the outlined strategic direction and vision. This may help support the CNS's decision to decline involvement in requests or readily accept them for the right reasons. Refer to Chapter 7, "Prioritizing: Avoiding Overcommitment and Under-achievement" for other strategies on this topic.

Professional Association Involvement

CNSs need the opportunity to meet, support, and share ideas with other CNS colleagues regularly. Involvement with CNSs locally in the area may be possible within your hospital or clinic setting or in the surrounding community, whether formally as a CNS Council or informally arranged by CNS colleagues with opportunities to meet as needed. Clinical specialty organizations may provide an opportunity to network with other CNS and RN colleagues both for clinical specialty and for CNS role development components.

Active involvement with the NACNS has provided a great deal of support for my role and growth as a CNS. Involvement in an NACNS committee and attending the annual NACNS conference each year are crucial priorities for networking with CNS colleagues at the conference and throughout the year via e-mail or phone, as desired. Graduate students should be encouraged to become involved with the professional nursing association for their clinical specialty and for CNS role development, they should become active members of NACNS to be well-rounded CNSs. Additional discussion of this topic is featured in Chapter 15, "Becoming Involved With Professional Organizations."

Evaluation of the Clinical Partnership/Experience

At the end of the clinical preceptorship with the CNS graduate student, an evaluation is done of the achievement of planned goals, objectives, and student performance overall. This formal, written evaluation is supplied by the graduate student/ program, often at the beginning of the clinical preceptorship. The tool should be reviewed together in the initial goal-planning stage and agreed upon as the evaluation that will be utilized to provide feedback. Sharing the completed evaluation or completing it with the CNS graduate student may provide for effective feedback, including highlights of strengths identified in performance and opportunities for growth and further development. Honest feedback from the CNS graduate student about the preceptorship experience at the facility and with you or others as CNS preceptor/mentor for appropriateness as a preceptor is also helpful for improvements for future CNS students (Stark, 2004). As RN and CNS colleagues, sharing this important information honestly and in a supportive manner is critically important for the growth of both persons. Mutual perceived achievement of assisting the CNS graduate student in progressing toward becoming a safe, competent, compassionate, innovative, and collaborative CNS clinician would be a great outcome for your clinical preceptorship together (Burns et al., 2006).

Conclusion

Serving as a preceptor to CNS graduate students has provided me with great professional and personal satisfaction over the years. By sharing with the new CNS colleague the successful CNS projects and strategies I have implemented, the times I have stumbled along the way, and lessons learned from all of these experiences, I feel I am helping shape the future of CNS practice and the great contributions that can be made by each of us. I have always felt committed to precept, mentor, and guide other professional colleagues as a way to thank and honor all those nursing professionals who helped me be the CNS I am today. Following a plan, such as those outlined in this chapter, helps to keep your focus as a CNS on your established priorities and contributions to outcomes for patients, nurses, and the organization. This also allows for proactive or strategic planning and may facilitate preserving some of your time so that there is opportunity to precept graduate CNS students and fully invite them into experiencing the CNS role. Much time and energy are often needed to precept students and can feel overwhelming with so many other demands for our time. Choosing our attitude as one of being positive and welcoming will greatly assist you and the CNS student in having a great experience together for the clinical preceptorship. I have learned that CNS students are eager to learn, appreciate your valuable time and the energy you invest in them, and can contribute much if you let them. I still use today in my CNS practice many of the ideas, projects, and other contributions that CNS graduate students developed during their clinical preceptorship. Many of these colleagues are successfully implementing their CNS roles in various settings and maintain a professional relationship with me. I enjoy every interaction I have with them and hope their experiences as CNS students helped shape their current practice and that they too will help share their knowledge and skills gained with other professional colleagues in the near future.

References

American Association of Colleges of Nursing. (2002, January). *AACN white paper: Hallmarks of the professional nursing practice environment.* Retrieved June 13, 2007, from http://www.aacn.nche.edu/publications/positions/hallmarks.htm

Brown, Y. (2007). Staff development story. *Journal for Nurses in Staff Development* (Sept/Oct), 243–245.

Burns, C., Beauchesne, M., Ryan-Krause, P., & Sawin, K. (2006). Mastering the preceptor role: Challenges of clinical thinking. *Journal of Pediatric Health Care, 20*(3), 172–183.

Butler, M., & Felts, J. (2006). Tool kit for the staff mentor: Strategies for improving retention. *The Journal of Continuing Education in Nursing, 37*(5), 210–213.

Campbell, G. (2006, March 16). "Defining success in the CNS role: An administrative perspective." Presented at the NACNS Annual Conference, March 15–18, 2006, Salt Lake City, Utah.

Firtko, A., Stewart, R., & Knox, N. (2005). Understanding mentoring and preceptorship: Clarifying the quagmire. *Contemporary Nurse, 19*(1–2), 32–40.

Modic, M., & Harris, R. (2007). Mastering precepting: Using the BECOME method to enhance clinical thinking. *Journal for Nurses in Staff Development, 23*(1), 1–9.

Myrick, F., & Yonge, O. (2004). Enhancing critical thinking in the preceptorship experience in nursing education. *Journal of Advanced Nursing, 45*(4), 371–380.

National Association of Clinical Nurse Specialists (NACNS). (2004). *Statement on clinical nurse specialist practice and education* (2nd ed.). Harrisburg, PA: Author.

Stark, S. (2004). Preceptor's expectations: An avenue to foster appropriate clinical experiences for advanced practice nursing students. *The Journal of Continuing Education in Nursing, 35*(5), 234–235.

IV

Evaluation

13

Documenting Clinical Outcomes

Deborah G. Klein

Increased demand for accountability, ongoing changes in health care delivery, and changing reimbursement have pushed clinical nurse specialists (CNSs) to verify their contributions and demonstrate their value. CNSs are becoming more involved in collecting and using clinical, economic, and quality outcomes data. Evidence of CNS impact occurs in many ways, including outcome measurement activities, process improvement analysis, and program evaluation. *Statement on Clinical Nurse Specialist Practice and Education* (National Association of Clinical Nurse Specialists [NACNS], 2004) outlines core competencies and essential characteristics of CNS practice that produce outcomes. Achievement of these outcomes is driven by individual interest, availability of financial and material resources, expectations of the institution, organizational culture, and support of others. Even the new CNS must consider ways to demonstrate impact on clinical outcomes.

The new CNS must often demonstrate that one is a clinical expert before one can impact clinical outcomes (Klein, 2007). However, with strong clinical leadership skills, including open-mindedness, professional demeanor, mentoring, and excellent communication skills, a new CNS can impact clinical outcomes while demonstrating clinical expertise. The ability of the CNS to

13.1 Outcome Evaluation Planning Process

Phase I: Define the Core Question
1. Clarify the question
2. Define the population to be evaluated
3. Identify the stakeholders
4. Review the literature
5. Identify interventions
6. Develop the core question

Phase II: Define the Data Elements
1. Identify the population
2. Establish performance and outcome measures or indicators
3. Identify and evaluate the data

Phase III: Derive Meaning From Data and Act on Results
1. Analyze data and interpret results
2. Present and disseminate findings
3. Identify improvement opportunities
4. Develop a plan for implementation and reevaluate

Adapted from Ingersoll and Mahn-DiNicola (2005).

recognize patterns in resource utilization and care delivery processes makes the CNS an ideal facilitator of quality improvement activities in which data can direct and support decisions on how to achieve best practices (Duffy, 2002; Ingersoll & Mahn-DiNicola, 2005). System inefficiencies, obstacles to continuity of care, and the inability of others to see the "big picture" can be identified through pattern recognition.

Three phases have been described that serve as a framework for the development of an effective outcome evaluation plan that any CNS can use (Ingersoll & Mahn-DiNicola, 2005). The first phase is defining the core questions that need to be answered; the second phase is defining the data required to answer the questions; and the third phase focuses on deriving meaning from the data and acting on the result (Box 13.1).

Define the Core Question

Defining the core question is the foundation for developing an effective outcome plan. As part of this process the CNS must ensure that the question clarifies the purpose and the goals of the CNS within the organization. The CNS should discuss with the nurse manager or administrator the role expectations to ensure that they are reasonable and appropriate. Attempts should be made to focus on nurse-sensitive outcomes (patient falls, ventilator-associated pneumonia, skin breakdown) rather than areas where the CNS may have an impact (decreasing length of stay, decreasing hospital costs). The new CNS must ensure that the question is simple and able to be successfully answered. By successfully addressing a clinical practice concern, the new CNS will gain credibility and respect.

Questions can come from CNS observations of clinical practice, quality data, or directly from the nursing staff. The nurse manager may approach the new CNS with a clinical issue that needs further development, for example, strategies to reduce patient falls, effectiveness of pain management, evaluating documentation of restraints, or examining skin breakdown rates. Although the new CNS may not desire to focus on these issues, selecting one of these areas for process improvement is an effective way to demonstrate cooperation, collaboration, and credibility, and to earn trust and respect.

One of the most important areas in which the CNS has value is in helping to ensure that evidence-based practice changes are implemented. Several national quality and safety measures have been published that focus on high-volume, high-risk populations that can serve as guides for developing CNS outcome evaluation plans. Some of these measures include the 2007 National Patient Safety Goals from the Joint Commission, National Quality Improvement Goals—Oryx Performance Core Measures from the Joint Commission, National Quality Forum, Agency for Healthcare Research and Quality of the Department of Health and Human Services, Institute of Medicine's 5 Million Lives Campaign, Surviving Sepsis Campaign, and The Leapfrog Safe Practices Score. The new CNS can refer to any one of these sources for identifying potential questions.

The next step is to define the population to be evaluated. Many CNSs use a variety of activities with heterogeneous populations in their clinical practice. Therefore, it is necessary for the CNS to focus on specific aspects of practice with a specific patient group. This focus helps create a more manageable and successful outcome plan and limits extraneous variables that could interfere with the interpretation of the findings. For example, the new CNS should consider limiting the population to one unit (surgical intensive care unit) or a specific aspect of a diagnosis (diabetic patients with foot ulcers seen in an outpatient clinic). If possible, the target population should be comparable to other groups monitored through quality improvement activities at the organizational or department level.

The CNS must also identify the stakeholders in the process. The CNS is often the individual facilitating the team, and early identification of the stakeholders will facilitate the design of the outcome evaluation. Stakeholders may include nursing staff, nurse manager, physicians, pharmacists, and other members of the health care team. Encouraging their participation early on, incorporating their ideas, and providing updates throughout the process will help clarify the CNS role to them and acknowledge the new CNS as a valuable member of the team. Together these individuals become the process team.

The nurse manager of the patient care area is responsible for ensuring that the unit has the needed resources, that staff have the necessary skills and knowledge to perform their jobs, and that the environment supports the staff in delivering care and meeting organizational goals (Disch, Walton, & Barnsteiner, 2001). The CNS can support these nurse manager responsibilities, and together the CNS and the nurse manager can develop a strong partnership in ensuring that nursing standards form the basis of nursing practice. It is imperative that

13.2   Questions That Can Be Used in Creating an Outcome Evaluation Plan

How cost effective is this program?
How satisfied are patients with the service they receive?
How closely does the health care team adhere to best-practice standards?
What are the barriers that influence the ability of the staff to carry out the practice?
How many patients have complications of care?
What patient safety issues associated with this population should we examine?
What can be done to reduce resource utilization for this population?
What do we need to do differently to become a center of excellence for this population?
How can the CNS contribute to the training and development of other staff?

Adapted from Ingersoll and Mahn-DiNicola (2005) and Gawlinski (2007).

the nurse manager support the outcome evaluation plan. Not only will the CNS benefit, but the desired outcomes will impact nursing practice on that unit. In many instances, it may be the nurse manager who identifies an outcome project for the new CNS.

The final step is to review the literature for current standards of care, regulatory requirements, national guidelines, and established or emerging evidence-based best practices that are relevant to the question. Outcome data already available in an institution should also be considered, as this will save time, energy, and money (Gawlinski, 2007). Using this information, interventions can be identified. These interventions may include a new documentation tool, patient education materials, or the development of a new process to ensure patient safety. Once goals and interventions are identified, the core question can be developed. Ingersoll and Mahn-DiNicola (2005) have formulated some basic questions that can be useful to ask to help establish the outcome evaluation plan (Box 13.2). Once the core questions are determined by the CNS and other members of the process team, the data collection method can be designed.

Define the Data Elements

There are three steps in defining the data elements: identify the population, establish performance and outcome measures or indicators, and identify and evaluate the data. This phase is often challenging for the new CNS, particularly if the CNS has had little exposure to quality improvement principles and management information systems, both of which support outcome evaluation. The CNS should seek assistance from other health care professionals who have experience in continuous quality improvement principles, health care statistics, nursing informatics, or program evaluation.

Although identifying the population may seem obvious, it is important to determine inclusion criteria. This will serve as the denominator for the specific indicator, which is typically a number, rate, or sum. For example, it may be easier to study interventions that decrease the incidence of ventilator-associated pneumonia in intubated patients on mechanical ventilation in *one* intensive care unit (ICU) as the target population than to include all intubated patients on mechanical ventilation in *several* ICUs.

Establishing performance and outcome measures or indicators involves determining which data will be collected to answer the core question. The CNS should consider data available from national database services for benchmarking. Indicators can include readmission rates for a specific diagnosis, patient falls rate per 1,000 patient days, central line infections per 1,000 line days, or average length of stay. A draft list of indicators should be created and shared with the team for feedback and suggestions. Achieving team support of the indicators is imperative for the CNS to be perceived as being able to successfully answer the core question and therefore be effective in the CNS role.

The new CNS must be aware that one may be asked to collect data for other health care providers that have little to do with the CNS's ability to influence care. For example, interventional cardiologists are interested in the time from the first incision for patients undergoing stent placement to the time the wire crosses the lesion in the coronary artery. The CNS has no role in influencing this process, and it should not be part of a CNS outcome plan. The CNS can, however, identify other potential resources that may be available to gather this information. The CNS must stay focused on goals for which one is responsible.

The final step is identifying and evaluating the data elements. A new CNS may consider using short-term outcome measures, such as blood glucose levels, pressure ulcer development, or patient falls, instead of long-term outcomes measures, such as readmission rates, return clinic visits, or length of stay (Byers & Brunell, 1998). The details of the data collection tools and the actual data collection process are examined. How easy is the instrument to use? How much time does it take to complete? Is this tool useful in determining the effect of the CNS in nursing practice? Whenever possible, it is easier to use instruments already established rather than develop new ones. The data collection instrument should be short, concise, user-friendly, and easy to complete.

To help the CNS determine which indicators are essential versus those that are interesting but not essential, the CNS can list each indicator on a piece of paper and then write down all aspects of data collection for each indicator. For example, if determining a rate, definitions of the numerator and denominator and the source for each data element are listed. Hospital management information systems can be a source of data. Risk management systems can provide details of medication errors, transfusion reactions, or other adverse outcomes. Pharmacy systems may track the time when first dose of a specific medication was administered or the number of doses of a specific medication a patient received. Laboratory, radiology, and clinical documentation systems can also provide needed data. Experts are available to assist in retrieving data from these systems.

Outcome indicators should be measured before (at baseline) and after the practice change. Measurement at these times allows a before and after comparison of the effects of the practice change.

Once the indicators and data elements have been finalized and the data sources determined, the CNS should summarize the outcome evaluation plan in a concise document. Timelines and who is responsible for data collection and data analysis are included. Documenting the plan in this manner simplifies implementation and clarifies the responsibility of all participants. This document is shared with the process team to ensure support.

Derive Meaning From Data and Act on Results

The final phase of the outcome evaluation plan process includes analyzing, evaluating, and disseminating the findings, along with identifying opportunities for improvement. The goal is to improve quality, cost, and customer satisfaction, and to evaluate the contributions of the CNS.

The CNS may be responsible for data analysis; however, including others (statistician or doctorally prepared nurse researcher) in the process may help eliminate any perceived bias. The resulting data can be compared with baseline information or a known standard of care or benchmark.

Findings, conclusions, and recommendations for future practice are essential components of the outcome evaluation process. The way the findings are presented will depend on the personnel receiving the information. Generally, charts or tables are an effective way to present data. Control charts display performance data against upper and lower control limits that reflect normal variation in a system. Data lying outside the upper and lower limits and clusters of data within the limits indicate variations that require further investigation.

Control charts can also document processes over time. For example, it was noted that despite the implementation of an insulin infusion protocol and preprinted order set in an ICU, blood glucose levels were not within the expected range 60% of the time. The CNS led a team of staff nurses, nurse manager, pharmacist, and the medical director of the ICU in developing and implementing a process to move blood glucose levels into the expected range. Data for the control chart were used to show meaningful changes that occurred as a result of the CNS's efforts (Figure 13.1). The longitudinal display of data provides an accurate and informative representation of the CNS impact than would be seen by a simple comparison of average blood glucose levels before and after the intervention.

Once the findings have been prepared for review, they must be interpreted and potential opportunities for improvement identified. This process is similar to any work design initiative. Champions and potential opponents of change should be identified. Specific goals and interventions are developed as well as the level of difficulty with implementing the change, projected costs, and the human and technological resources required to implement and sustain the change. The CNS must consider how much time will be involved in this project and how it may affect other areas of practice. For example, if the goal of the performance improvement plan is to maintain the patient's blood glucose levels between 80 mg/dl and 120 mg/dl, interventions might include reeducating the nursing staff in the ICU on the insulin infusion protocol to ensure that it is initiated at the appropriate time. Although the time commitment to review the insulin infusion protocol with 60 RNs will be great, the benefit to the patient will be even greater. In addition, it will help establish credibility for the new CNS.

Once goals and strategies to meet these goals have been established, they should be summarized and distributed to the process team as well as to the

13.1

Blood glucose levels using insulin infusion protocol control chart.

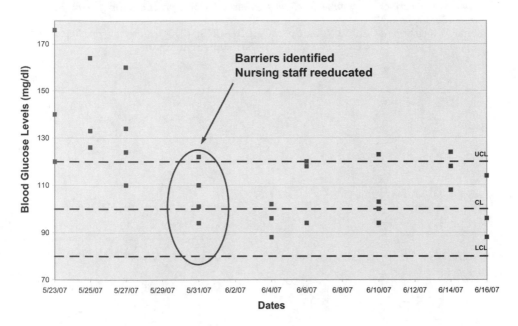

nursing staff and attendees of department meetings. Each goal should specify the primary intervention that will be used to reach the goal as well as who is accountable for the actions required and the target dates for completion. The CNS can then use this established plan to reevaluate the outcome, which can then be used as the basis for future outcome evaluation plans. Other strategies to ensure that practice changes are sustained include incorporating them into institutional documents such as policies, procedures, guidelines, and competencies as well as orientation programs.

Documenting clinical outcomes is a challenge for a new CNS. However, by identifying a simple clinical question, acknowledging the stakeholders and listening to their ideas, reviewing the literature, defining the population, establishing the outcome indicators, collecting and analyzing the data, interpreting the results, presenting the results with a plan for implementing changes, and implementing the plan, the CNS can successfully demonstrate one's value.

References

Byers, J. F., & Brunell, M. L. (1998). Demonstrating the value of the advanced practice nurse: An evaluation model. *AACN Clinical Issues: Advanced Practice in Acute and Critical Care, 9,* 296–305.

Disch, J., Walton, M., & Barnsteiner, J. (2001). The role of the clinical nurse specialist in creating a healthy work environment. *AACN Clinical Issues: Advanced Practice in Acute and Critical Care, 12,* 345–355.

Duffy, J. R. (2002). The clinical leadership role of the CNS in the identification of nurse-sensitive and multidisciplinary quality indicator sets. *Clinical Nurse Specialist, 16,* 70–76.

Gawlinski, A. (2007). Evidence-based practice changes: Measuring the outcome. *AACN Advanced Critical Care, 18,* 320–322.

Ingersoll, G. L., & Mahn-DiNicola, V. A. (2005). Outcome evaluation and performance improvement. In A. Hamric, J. A. Spross, & C. M. Hanson (Eds.), *Advanced practice nursing: An
   integrative approach* (pp. 875–941). St Louis: Saunders Elsevier.
Klein, D. G. (2007). From novice to expert: CNS competencies. In M. McKinley (Ed.), *Acute
   and critical care clinical nurse specialists: Synergy for best practices* (pp. 11–28). St Louis:
   Saunders Elsevier.
National Association of Clinical Nurse Specialists (NACNS). (2004). *Statement on clinical nurse
   specialist practice and education* (2nd ed.). Harrisburg, PA: Author.

14

Communicating Results: Who Needs to Know What

Kathy Wright

The role of the clinical nurse specialist (CNS) can provide a unique and measurable impact upon the patient/client, nursing personnel, and organizations/networks. The CNS's ongoing acquisition of current evidence-based knowledge and skills facilitates positive outcomes across all three spheres of influence. The CNS must be a skilled communicator to most effectively influence and inspire others. Basic yet effective interpersonal skills include reflection or validating communication received from others, providing constructive feedback, conveying a caring attitude, and lastly, formulating and logically conveying ideas, all the while being sensitive to the needs and feelings of others (National Association of Clinical Nurse Specialists [NACNS], 2004).

In each sphere of influence, the sharing of significant information facilitates positive outcomes in areas such as complex patient management, nursing practice/performance parameters, policy/program development, or best-practice care guidelines. When communicating with others, it is important to address the recipient's behavioral style. Many individuals have described different recognizable traits to address preferred communication styles. Ron Willingham (2003), a customer service specialist, describes a behavioral styles model with four different personality types that range from process-oriented to results-oriented. Process-oriented communicators include:

- Talkers—who are friendly and want to connect on a personal level; less interested in details than they are in social approval and acceptance; and prefer a collaborative approach to decision making and problem solving.
- Supporters—similarly relationship-oriented, but are detail-minded, easygoing, and dependable; they need time to process information and cannot be pressed for a quick decision.

On the results-oriented end of the spectrum, Willingham describes the "doers" and the "controllers":

- Doers—get to the point and make decisions quickly; action-oriented and less concerned with relationships, they expect to deal with the "top person" and want recognition for their achievements.
- Controllers—need for extensive factual information or data; well-organized and detail-oriented, they are most easily recognized by their low, reserved emotional tone and need to weigh all alternatives before making a decision.

A team approach works most effectively with a balance of different styles, as each brings different strengths to the work to be accomplished; no one style is better or more suited to the CNS role than another. Often people are a combination of two or even three styles. It will be helpful, however, for the CNS to recognize personal behavioral style and to recognize the styles of those with whom communication occurs; rapport may be established more quickly and communication flow more smoothly when attempts are made to match the style of those with whom communication is needed in the three spheres of CNS influence.

Spheres of Influence

Patients/Clients

The CNS facilitates integration of a high-level, holistic assessment and treatment plan toward optimal disease management or wellness. Prevention, alleviation, and/or reduction of risky behavior can be achieved with innovative educational programs. The most effective communication with patients or clients, and associated significant others, is geared to the appropriate level of education and preferred learning style. Printed teaching materials should be written at a 4th to 6th grade reading level. The CNS can utilize computer-based tools to ensure that sentence structure and vocabulary are conducive to the consumer's comprehension. The CNS should ask the learner how the information will be best absorbed and retained—written material, verbal instruction, or demonstration; observation of the learner's assimilation of material taught will further confirm the best teaching methodology. Printed teaching materials, individualized to address specific patient needs and to include the CNS's contact information for future reference, serve as valuable tools in promoting continuity of care.

Coordination of patient/client care to maximize use of available organizational and/or community resources is an important aspect of the CNS role, as is the coordination of transitions across the care continuum. Patients/families who understand the specifics related to their health care can often provide a vital communication link as the care setting changes. When patients and their families are informed of their role in the health care journey and given appropriate information to ease transitions and challenges, the outcomes are more likely to be positive.

Nursing Personnel

As a consultant or mentor, the CNS has the potential to significantly impact nursing personnel and other care providers. In day-to-day communications with physicians and others within the health care team, the message must be clear and concise. Many facilities utilize the SBAR (situation, background, assessment, and recommendation) format to facilitate this process:

- *Situation*—a one-line statement indicating phenomena of concern, for example, "I am calling about . . ."
- *Background*—subjective and objective data related to the situation, for example, "The patient is agitated and confused . . ."
- *Assessment*—what is suspected as problematic, for example, "The problem seems to be . . ."
- *Recommendation*—what is suggested as a solution or plan, for example, "I suggest that you . . ."

The SBAR communication technique was developed by the armed forces years ago and initially adapted for use between health care providers by Michael Leonard, MD, Physician Leader for Patient Safety at Kaiser Permanente, along with colleagues Doug Bonacum and Suzanne Graham at Kaiser Permanente of Evergreen, Colorado. Use of the SBAR technique facilitates an effective verbal exchange of information between care providers, or it can be used in a written format to allow care providers to communicate a request for a physician's order specific to an identified patient need (Institute for Healthcare Improvement, 2007).

Frequently, the CNS will be called upon to facilitate changes in clinical practice. The change process is facilitated when staff members are encouraged to participate in creating solutions. Collaboration with others toward common goals must include recognition and acceptance of the separate and combined skill sets, and areas of responsibility, along with mutual safeguarding of the legitimate interests of each party. In the book *Crucial Conversations: Tools for Talking When the Stakes Are High* (Patterson, Grenny, McMillan, & Switler, 2002), the reader is encouraged to "CRIB":

- Commit to seek a common purpose—staying in the conversation until common ground is identified.

■ Recognize the purpose behind the strategy—separate demands from the purpose they might serve.

■ Invent a mutual purpose—reach beyond the multiple agendas from individuals and sometimes a long-term goal will take all involved to a higher level.

■ Brainstorm new strategies—be open to everyone's ideas and the group might be surprised at the teamwork that evolves!

A relationship of trust with the CNS and nursing leadership will enhance the nursing staff's comfort with the ambiguity and uncertainty sometimes associated with the journey. Schultz (2007) describes the diffusion of innovation theory in four stages, including knowledge, persuasion, decision, and finally, staff engagement. In the implementation of evidence-based practice, identification of learning needs or gaps in knowledge, skills, and competencies related to change can effectively trigger solutions via classroom education, skills labs, or on-the-unit mentorship. The associated self-mastery will increase staff's capacity to manage their fear of change, while increasing their ability to support and encourage others (Viney & Rivers, 2007).

Organizations/Networks

As a CNS functions within organizations or networks, communication of crucial information to key players is essential. Some of the critical information to be shared will relate to fundamental topics such as safety, quality, and productivity; additionally, discussions on change management, teamwork, and innovations in clinical practice set the CNS apart as a forward-thinking leader.

For example, organizational budget crunches regularly cause employers to closely examine distribution of available resources. The CNS may find it helpful to keep a monthly tally to reflect productivity. It is very important that direct care/patient volume statistics not be the sole indicator of the CNS's workload. Other critical CNS activities, such as staff education, performance improvement projects, research/publication, and committee meetings, should be made visible. See Table 14.1, developed and utilized by the author in her wound, ostomy, and continence CNS role. In order to collate such data, a spreadsheet for daily capture of this information was established, as was a report for comparison of annual totals.

CNS competencies fulfill organizational needs for a leader who can design evidence-based care guidelines for specific patient populations. Identification of patterns within a population or system will facilitate recognition of what is working well, what needs to be fixed, and what interventions will result most consistently in quality patient outcomes. Real or near-miss consequences and errors in patient care across the organization must be tracked, reported, and managed. Consistency in format for reporting of performance improvement activities ensures that vital components will not be omitted. The author developed a suggested report format, which has been disseminated by her employer for organization-wide use (see Table 14.2). A graph reflecting a specific unit's progress or comparing units across the organization can be posted to communicate results of staff efforts and stimulate dialogue.

14.1 Wound, Ostomy, and Continence Clinical Nurse Specialist Reporting Statistics

WOC STATS	Jan	Feb	March	April	May	June	July	Aug	Sept	Oct	Nov	Dec	TOTAL
TOTAL VISITS													
Inpatient													
ECF													
Home													
Outpatient													
Total pts													
Inpatient													
LTC													
Home													
Outpatient													
Inpatient hours													
Contracted hrs													
Noncharged hrs													
CASE MIX													
Ostomy													
Preventive													
PU													

(Continued)

14.1 Wound, Ostomy, and Continence Clinical Nurse Specialist Reporting Statistics (*Continued*)

WOC STATS	Jan	Feb	March	April	May	June	July	Aug	Sept	Oct	Nov	Dec	TOTAL
Draining wound													
Fistulas													
ACQUIRED PU													
ICU													
PCU													
MS													
Peds/SSU													
ER													
LTC													
1st													
2nd													
CNS FUNCTIONS													
Staff education													
Admin/office time													
Meetings													
Research													
Publication													
Perf improvement													

14.2	**Performance Improvement Report**

I.   Date:

II. Month of data collection:

III. Submitted by:

IV. Data collected by:

V.   Purpose of study/audit:

VI. Sample size:

VII. Criteria monitored: (Attach audit tool, if appropriate)

VIII. Data summation/Analysis: (Attach illustrative graph/pie chart)

IX. Recommendations/Actions:

Arellano and Bennet (2007) recommend use of the "4 Ds" by nursing leaders in ensuring regulatory survey readiness and facilitating the provision of high-quality patient care:

- Define policies and procedures that are both realistic and reflective of current standards of practice and regulatory guidelines.
- Develop systems and processes to support communication to the care provider level on policy and procedure changes, and to ensure accountability for implementation.
- Deliver patient care reflective of compliance with the defined policies and procedures.
- Document in a concise, consistent, and effective manner.

An appropriate ending for a chapter on communication is a reminder that effective listening is an essential communication skill for the CNS, no matter in which sphere of influence the exchange is occurring. In the busy pace of the CNS's workday, it is all too easy to get caught up in the *tasks* to be completed and lose sight of the *people* to be served. Focusing on the moment, tuning out multiple distracters, and being truly present in every exchange will facilitate the most effective communication and bring the CNS greater role success and satisfaction!

References

Arellano, M., & Bennet, J. (2007). Ensuring survey readiness every day. *Extended Care Product News,* July/August, 13–14.

Institute for Healthcare Improvement. (2007). SBAR technique for communication: A situational briefing. Retrieved November 16, 2008, from http://www.ihi.org/IHI/Topics /PatientSafety/ SafetyGeneral/Tools/SBARTechniqueforCommunicationASituationalBriefingModel.htm

National Association of Clinical Nurse Specialists (NACNS). (2004). *Statement on clinical nurse specialist practice and education* (2nd ed.). Harrisburg, PA: Author.

Patterson, K., Grenny, J., McMillan, R., & Switler, A. (2002). *Crucial conversations: Tools for talking when the stakes are high.* New York: McGraw Hill.

Schultz, A. (2007). Implementation: A team effort. *Nursing Management,* June, 10–14.

Viney, M., & Rivers, N. (2007). Frontline managers lead an innovative improvement model. *Nursing Management,* June, 10–14.

Willingham, R. (2003). *Integrity selling for the 21st century.* New York: Doubleday.

V

Reaching Out

15

Becoming Involved With Professional Organizations

Mary Fran Tracy

Patrick Schultz

As you are embarking on a new career as a clinical nurse specialist (CNS), it may seem overwhelming to even consider getting involved in professional organizations as well. However, involvement in professional organizations may actually offer you a number of resource and networking opportunities and facilitate transition into your new role. Although active involvement may not be feasible right away, it is important to consider how simply being a member of a professional organization can benefit you as a new CNS. In addition, it may be helpful to keep in mind a target timeline for increasing professional involvement as a goal toward which to strive.

There can be many benefits of belonging to and being active in a professional organization. Getting involved in professional organizations as a CNS can result in advancement of the profession of nursing, promotion of self-development, and ultimately improvement of patient care. With over 70 nursing organizations to choose from, in addition to other multidisciplinary and professional organizations, there are multiple options to find an organization that matches your needs. This chapter will give you ideas to consider related to this aspect of your career.

Choosing an Organization

If you were active in professional organizations prior to becoming a CNS, you may already be familiar with existing professional organizations. However, as a CNS student and novice CNS, you may now have different professional needs. This is a great time to explore other organizations! CNSs frequently belong to more than one professional organization. Organizations attract different members because they exist for different purposes. Some organizations are structured to meet the needs of nurses caring for certain patient populations, while some focus on nurses in certain roles. An organization may exist for a single profession, while other organizations are multidisciplinary (see Table 15.1).

What should you look for when you are deciding to join a professional organization and considering becoming actively in/volved? Going to the organization's Web site can give you insight into the organization—its focus and priorities. Typically an organization will display its mission and vision on its Web site. Reviewing these statements should give you an overall view of the

15.1 Examples of Professional Organizations

Organization Type	Web Site
Profession-Based Organizations	
• American Nurses Association (ANA)	http://nursingworld.org/
• State-based ANA Organizations	http://nursingworld.org/ (constituent member associations)
Multidisciplinary Organizations	
• Society of Critical Care Medicine (SCCM)	http://www.sccm.org/
• American Heart Association (AHA)	https://www.americanheart.org/
• American Diabetes Association (ADA)	http://www.diabetes.org/
Role-Based Organizations	
• National Association of Clinical Nurse Specialists (NACNS)	http://www.nacns.org/
• National Nursing Staff Development Organization (NNSDO)	https://www.nnsdo.org/
• American Organization of Nurse Executives (AONE)	http://www.aone.org/
Population-Based Nursing Organizations	
• American Association of Critical-Care Nurses (AACN)	http://www.aacn.org/
• Oncology Nursing Society (ONS)	http://www.ons.org/
• Wound, Ostomy, and Continence Nurses Society (WOCN)	http://www.wocn.org/
• American Psychiatric Nurses Association (APNA)	http://www.apna.org/
• Association of periOperative Registered Nurses (AORN)	http://www.aorn.org/

15.1   Potential Membership Benefits

- Journal subscriptions
- Newsletters
- Networking opportunities—internal and external to organization
- "Representing your voice"
- Listserv participation
- Reduced rates for insurance or other group benefits
- Reduced rates for certification examinations
- Reduced registration fees to sponsored conferences
- Reduced rates for purchase of products
- Volunteer opportunities
- Continuing education opportunities
- Participation in a community of practice

organization and its stated purpose for existing. Reviewing this information can give you a quick glimpse at the alignment of an organization with your goals and expectations as a member.

Reviewing other aspects of the organizational structure will give further insight into alignment: What are the organization's priorities? Do they match your expectations of how your dues would be spent? What is the leadership structure and how diverse are the leaders? Is it only a national organization, or does it have a local, state, or regional structure as well? How long has the organization been in existence, and what are the demographics of its members? Exploring these questions can help you decide whether a particular organization meets your needs and expectations.

Web sites may display a great deal of additional information and can be good resources, whether you actually join the organization as a member or simply use the resources in your CNS role. Many organizations post listings of educational offerings, organizational position statements, products for sale, and free resources on their Web page. Web sites will also typically list the cost of membership dues and the benefits that come with membership (see Box 15.1). While the actual amount of dues is a significant piece of information, it is also important to consider the monetary value of membership in context with the benefits—both tangible and intangible—of being a member.

Benefits of Professional Organization Membership and Involvement

Keeping Informed

A major benefit of membership is the opportunity for staying updated in your area of specialty or interest. Many organizations publish journals or newsletters with the latest information. For a nursing organization with a clinical focus, journals frequently provide the latest practice developments and an opportunity to see how others are providing care for similar populations. Many organizations also provide content for continuing education in a variety of formats and fees. This is particularly important as you maintain requirements for your licensure and certifications. For organizations that are more role or profession focused, journals or newsletters may give updates on issues affecting your practice itself. Examples of this may include legislative activities that impact licensing or reimbursement, or activities impacting changes in professional standards.

Networking

Belonging to a professional organization is a great way to develop networks with colleagues who share your area of expertise or interest, both locally and across the country. Maybe you are the only CNS in your specialty in your setting. Or perhaps you are literally the only CNS! Connecting with colleagues can reassure you that you are not alone in the challenges you are facing. It can connect you with colleague resources that you may not have known existed, even in your own immediate geographic area. Becoming involved can provide a reservoir of resources to tap into when needed. It can provide a mechanism to broaden your perspective and help you see solutions or opportunities that you may not have recognized. These networking opportunities can present themselves through subscribing to member Listservs, networking at organizational conferences, and contacting organizational staff who can assist with helpful resources and contacts.

Connecting with colleagues can also offer insight into how other CNSs practice and how other CNS roles are structured. This can be valuable as you are developing in your own role and establishing your practice. Many new CNSs are interested in finding a mentor to help them as they begin their new career. Conversely, many experienced CNSs are committed to mentoring and fostering the development of novice CNSs. Involvement in an organization may help you find a colleague who would be a match as a mentor in the areas you are seeking to develop.

Opportunities for Professional Development

Activity in a professional organization can provide opportunities to develop leadership skills such as participating in and leading committees, helping groups come to consensus, and working on projects in a broader environment outside of work. As organizations are usually a mix of diverse members and perspectives, it is not uncommon when these diverse opinions lead to disagreements about actions or directions that should be taken. This creates an environment for you to develop and refine skills such as negotiation and conflict resolution, whether as an active member or as an organizational leader.

Many professional organizations are committed to providing education for their members. If you are interested in developing your presentation skills, you could offer to provide presentations at local or regional conferences. You may consider submitting abstracts for presentation at national conferences. You may also decide to develop your written communication skills by writing organizational newsletters or journals. Some organizations have created mentoring programs to partner nurses who are novices in these skills with more experienced nurses to co-present or co-author.

Being a Role Model for Staff

An important role that should not be neglected is that of being an example for staff. A CNS's membership and involvement in professional organizations is a great role model for the staff the CNS works with. Their involvement as members or certificants will give them benefits similar to yours. The successful CNS is one who enables staff to independently look at evidence for best practice. Membership can provide staff with resources that are evidence-based and can support them in critically evaluating their practice. In addition, your role modeling helps create enthusiasm and cohesiveness as a profession. A deeper collegial relationship is often formed between members of the same organization.

Contributing to the Profession

Belonging to and being active in professional organizations not only benefits you but also benefits the profession of nursing. Organizations advance the profession of nursing by generating and capitalizing on financial power, political power, and intellectual power through their membership. Your membership dues help generate financial power, which allows for strategic investments. Strategic investments can include research funds to advance the science of nursing and improve patient care, political investments that can impact advancements in the profession that affect your practice, and investments in nurses that can offer access to professional growth opportunities.

Political power is generated by unifying nurses throughout districts, states, regions, countries, and the world. As membership grows, so does the ability to influence legislators and stakeholders. Organizations develop positions based on the views of their members. As an active member you can use your professional organization to influence patient care and the nursing profession by making your views known. The organization has the strength and cohesiveness to augment the voices of members through advocacy and structure. In addition, as a member you may be able to take advantage of organizational resources on developing your own personal advocacy skills. Organizations have the resources to effect change that individual professionals may not be able to accomplish.

Intellectual power is generated by the coming together of diverse perspectives in nursing. Combining the thoughts of leaders from differing backgrounds, interests, and education can create formal or informal think tanks where unique solutions to problems and ideas for research and practice innovations can be generated. Having many perspectives can contribute to achieving goals as a group, whereas an individual working alone might not have such success. As a member, you benefit from facilitated access to these diverse colleagues.

The presence of nursing is established by the activities of professional organizations. They gather the attention of the media and the public. This is an important way for people to find out who nurses really are and what they really do. Stereotypes can be dismantled. Many organizations provide resources that you can use in your daily role to educate the public about what nurses and CNSs do. By attending meetings and networking with colleagues, you can showcase the CNS role to other nurses and professionals.

Professional nursing organizations give nurses the opportunity to stand alongside other professional organizations, thereby ensuring the nursing perspective is heard. By using your voice through your professional organization, you are influencing patient care and the nursing profession. Since membership organizations rely on knowing and meeting member needs, your needs can be addressed at the same time the needs of the nursing profession are addressed.

Getting Started

At this point, you hopefully realize the benefits for you and nursing by being involved in a professional organization. The first steps to investigating professional organizations to join may be triggered by a variety of reasons. As a CNS student looking toward graduation, exploring organizations that offer certification may be your first priority in connecting with an organization. Frequently, members of the affiliated organization pay a reduced fee to take the certification exam. As a new CNS, having access to journals and newsletters may be important. Reviewing journals in your institution's library will give you an idea about which organization memberships can provide you with a journal that can be valuable to you in your daily role. As mentioned previously, reviewing organizational information online will quickly give you perspective on what activities the organization is involved in and how the organization focuses its priorities. Attending either local or national conferences will give you a good sense for the organization, its fit for you, and opportunities for networking.

It may be easier to start organizational involvement at the local level. The organization's Web site will typically provide contact information on local, state, or regional chapters, offices, and Web sites. It is important to establish whether membership at a local level also requires membership at a national level. Find out the local meeting schedule and whether you need to be a member to attend or if you can attend either as a guest or for a fee. If you know a colleague who is a member, ask if you can attend an event to get to know the organization. It's easier to go with someone you know!

Volunteering

Once you decide to join an organization, don't be surprised if you are approached to volunteer for the organization. Resist the urge to assume you don't have the necessary skills to meet its needs! Consider how volunteering will fit within your professional and personal life. There are many ways to volunteer, and most organizations are willing to negotiate and utilize whatever you are able to offer. Consider offering to volunteer in ways that fit your time and lifestyle commitments. If you have a particular skill, it may be convenient to offer that skill in volunteering. Conversely, if you are looking to develop new skills and have the time to devote to that development, consider volunteering in an area that will be new and challenging for you with adequate support for development.

Most organizations have a variety of volunteer opportunities that can match your availability for time commitment. Don't hesitate to be clear about what you are able to offer in terms of time and commitment to ensure there is a match. Volunteer opportunities come in many different forms—from joining committees with face-to-face meetings, to performing volunteer work from home, to participating in a conference call to provide ideas or feedback. If you are interested in volunteering at the national level, most organizations will post a call for volunteers through their newsletters or Web sites. They may also maintain a member volunteer database, which is queried by the organization when a particular interest, skill, or volunteer commitment is needed. Regardless of how you choose to volunteer, carefully consider what you are committing to in order to avoid the unfortunate circumstance of having to withdraw at a later date due to an inability to follow through. Foremost, enjoy your volunteerism as an opportunity to broaden your horizons and acquire new collegial relationships that will enrich your professional career!

Conclusion

Inevitably you will be attracted to many different organizations for various personal reasons. Choosing the actual number of professional organizations you will join and in which you become an active member should be a thoughtful process. The process should include consideration of priorities, choosing an organization, and determining level of involvement.

First, evaluate your priority needs and interests. Those priorities will help you determine whether to choose a specialty population-related organization, a role-based organization, a multidisciplinary organization, or a profession-based organization. From those priorities, explore your options and choose one or more organizations to join.

Then, determine your level of involvement. Keep in mind your purpose for joining. As a novice CNS, be careful not to overextend yourself. A balance must be found between spending energy to become proficient in your new role and taking on more responsibility within professional organizations. However, the novice CNS must also be careful not to automatically say no to all new opportunities. It can be easy to think there is no time to become involved in the important work of professional organizations.

Finally, take time to evaluate how well your time and energy are being managed. Are you getting what you need out of your memberships? Are you able to honor your commitments adequately? As you develop in your role, you will continue to gain new perspectives on your professional needs, anticipating they will change over the course of your career. This may result in changes or additions to affiliations over time.

Transitioning to the CNS role can be challenging in and of itself, and it can be easy to defer joining and becoming an active member of professional organizations. However, becoming an active member of just one professional organization can provide innumerable opportunities for networking, professional development, and access to resources, which can be invaluable as a new CNS.

Additional Readings

Delesky, K. (2003). Factors affecting nurses' decisions to join and maintain membership in professional associations. *Journal of PeriAnesthesia Nursing, 18*(1), 8–17.

Foley, M. (2001). ANA: Preserving the core while preparing for the future. *American Nurse, 33*(2), 5.

Haylock, P. J. (2002). You and your professional organization. In D. J. Mason, J. K. Leavitt, & M. W. Chaffee (Eds.), *Policy and politics in nursing and health care* (pp. 609–620). St. Louis, MO: Saunders.

Shinn, L. (2002). Contemporary issues in professional organizations. In D. J. Mason, J. K. Leavitt, & M. W. Chaffee (Eds.), *Policy and politics in nursing and health care* (pp. 601–607). St. Louis, MO: Saunders.

White, M. J., & Olson, R. S. (2004). Factors affecting membership in specialty nursing organizations. *Rehabilitation Nursing, 29*(4), 131–137.

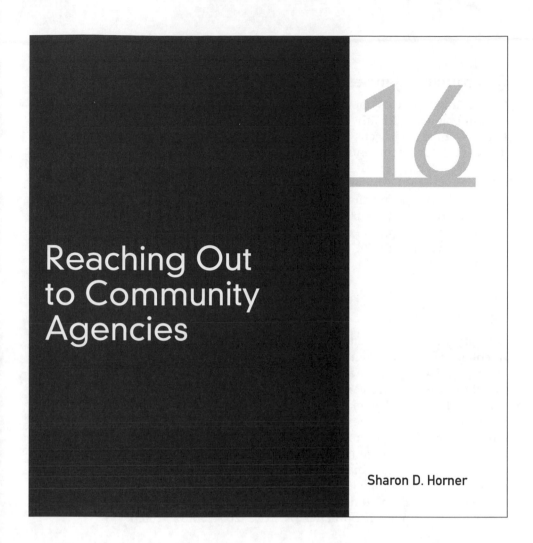

Reaching Out to Community Agencies

Sharon D. Horner

Americans have experienced significant health improvements over the preceding century, as evidenced by an increase in life span, greater control of communicable diseases, and reduction in mortality due to cardiovascular disease, stroke, and cancer (National Center for Health Statistics [NCHS], 2006). These health improvements have come about due to the integration of public health campaigns that promote healthy lifestyles with the careful application of therapeutic interventions to reduce or control health risks in at-risk populations. For example, lifestyle changes and the use of cholesterol- and hypertension-lowering medications in high-risk patients have significantly reduced mortality due to cardiovascular disease (NCHS, 2006). Clinical nurse specialists (CNSs) are well situated to build connections between acute care, chronic care, public health, and community organizations as they seek ways to improve the health of the clients they serve as well as the greater community. The focus of this chapter is on building collaborations with community agencies to extend the CNS's spheres of influence (National Association of Clinical Nurse Specialists [NACNS], 2004).

Community Agencies

Community agencies include entities that focus on physical health, social health, emotional health, and environmental health, as well as those that do not have an explicit focus on health. Many CNSs have had few opportunities to work with smaller community health-related agencies and likely no experience working with non-health-related community agencies during formal graduate school or even after graduation. Furthermore, since social service departments in health care organizations have established linkages with different community resources, the CNS may not appreciate the benefits of becoming involved with organizations in the community. Benefits of community collaboration can accrue to patients, to the community, to the institution that employs the CNS, and to the CNS.

Benefits to Patients

CNS practice is designed to improve patient-focused outcomes (NACNS, 2004). In collaboration with community agencies, the CNS can address health issues in the community that have the potential to improve patients' quality of life. Collaborative activities vary according to unique community needs but may include such activities as planning community-based health programs, conducting community assessments, creating resource banks (e.g., lending libraries, mobility aids) for community members, and testifying before health or governmental boards or committees. When health interventions are conceptualized on a continuum that ranges from primary prevention strategies (e.g., health promotion, health protection) to clinical therapeutic measures (e.g., secondary risk reduction, rehabilitation, palliation), community outreach can be seen as a natural extension of CNS practice (NACNS, 2004; Young, 2005).

Benefits to the Community

Effective strategies to address health needs and reduce health disparities within communities require collaboration among individuals, groups, and organizations (Collie-Akers et al., 2007). Community-based health programs need to address the physical, social, political, and economic factors that influence health care and health promotion activities.

A simple Google search yields a variety of community coalitions that have evolved to meet diverse communities' needs. Coalitions have been established to streamline fundraising activities for nonprofit organizations, balance economic growth while protecting the environment, raise the quality of life in a neighborhood or town, and target single issues such as long-term care, family violence, or networking with politicians. Many larger towns and cities have health-related coalitions that serve as mechanisms for the different, and sometimes competing, institutions to meet and work together on solving community-wide problems. When the CNS reaches out to community agencies, institutional and community agency resources can be leveraged to reach underserved populations or to tackle complex health issues that individual organizations alone would not be able to accomplish (Goddard, 2004).

Benefits to the Institution

The CNS's expertise is a valuable asset of the institution. When the CNS collaborates with community agencies on community health initiatives, this is a form of business philanthropy (Goddard, 2004). The institution is providing a major resource to the community without an expectation of gaining financial benefit. However, institutions generally require that such collaborations be consistent with the institutional mission and goals. While there is little-to-no expectation of financial gain, the institution should garner social benefits from such "good neighbor" collaborations.

Benefits to the CNS

The CNS can derive both professional and personal benefits by working with community agencies. Over time, as the CNS's expertise is recognized outside the institution, opportunities to contribute to a wide range of health-related issues will emerge. In turn, the CNS gains a sense of personal satisfaction as quality improvements are made available in the greater community.

Getting Started

The CNS should have a goal in mind when setting out to build connections with community agencies. Having a goal can help focus the CNS in identifying, contacting, and working with community agencies. For the CNS who is a novice or for the experienced CNS who is new to a community, the goal may simply be to identify the community resources available for a selected population and then to volunteer in community organizations that provide resources or services that are applicable to that population. Volunteering serves to introduce the CNS to community groups and is one means of building social capital (Goddard, 2004). For the established CNS who has developed or is developing programs of care for a selected population, the goal would most likely be focused on ways to extend the program of care into the community. A few examples of broadly defined community-based goals include reducing chronic diseases, improving the quality of life of persons with chronic conditions, or preventing injury and illness.

Identifying Community Agencies

Community health promotion interventions can be implemented by organized systems (e.g., community agencies, coalitions) or driven by grassroots efforts (e.g., neighborhood groups, community "watchdog" groups). In a study that examined 44 community health promotion interventions in European cities, all of the interventions involved collaborations between as few as 3 partners to as many as 1,700 partners, with 30 projects having formal collaborative structures (Sogoric, Middleton, Lang, Ivankovic, & Kern, 2005). Sogoric and colleagues found that interventions designed by health care systems were focused exclusively on physical health, while interventions designed by governments (e.g., town councils, county boards) also included social health and neighborhood health (Sogoric et al., 2005). They also found that interventions that were designed by health care organizations had the lowest involvement by community participants in the planning and evaluation of their programs when compared with local government health programs that had moderate community input. The highest input was provided in those programs designed by grassroots community groups. The programs that had moderate to high community input throughout the design and implementation of the projects had the greatest flexibility in responding to changing environmental conditions, whereas those programs that limited the participant input to "program satisfaction" had fixed structures and limited ability to respond to changing conditions. These findings support the need for CNSs to reach out to community agencies to develop health promotion interventions that are responsive to community-identified needs and adaptable to changing community conditions.

The CNS begins by identifying community agencies or coalitions whose mission or functional activities are congruent with the goal selected. For example, if the goal is to improve the quality of life for persons with a selected chronic condition, the CNS would identify agencies that serve the selected population, including formal organizations (e.g., American Heart Association, American Lung Association, American Cancer Society) and health care–based resources (e.g., Breast Cancer Support Group, Camp for All). However, the CNS should also look beyond these agencies to identify other groups or agencies that have the potential to contribute to quality of life in the realm of social or emotional functioning. For example, the community library may sponsor book clubs for groups with different interests, or a local specialty school (e.g., culinary or art school) might provide community classes that could be tailored to meet the needs of special groups. The inclusion of non-health-related agencies into a comprehensive health promotion initiative has the potential to yield important benefits to patients and the community partners.

Contacting Community Agencies

The CNS begins by gaining entrée into these community agencies (Yoo et al., 2003). Public agencies have newsletters or Web sites that explain missions and scopes of practice and provide lists of meetings and activities. The CNS can attend open meetings to learn more about the agency and to meet agency representatives. Because of their collaborative structure, community coalitions have meetings that are open to the community, making an easy point of entry for the CNS.

When the agency does not have open meetings, the CNS needs to establish entrée to the agency. Connections can be established through networking with colleagues (Rojas-Guyler, Murnan, & Cottrell, 2007). Networking can begin in the workplace as the CNS discusses his/her goals for community collaborations over lunch or before other institutional meetings. Established colleagues will offer advice and may have contacts with community agencies. Colleagues' introductions to community agency personnel can ease the CNS entrée into the agencies. The CNS also needs to attend professional meetings in the community to build collegial relationships outside the workplace, because representatives of community agencies may attend these local meetings. Such informal networking is a good way to begin reaching out to community agencies. Additionally, the CNS should view volunteering his/her services to support the agency's projects as a means of establishing connections with community agencies (Rojas-Guyler et al., 2007).

Working With Community Agencies

Community agencies have professional staff, non-professional support staff, and volunteers who work together to achieve the agency's mission and goals. This diverse mix of expertise and experience can be challenging when working with community agencies. At the same time it can be rewarding as one learns different ways of conceptualizing issues and different approaches to the same problem. Perhaps the most important rule is to *keep an open mind* when working with community agencies, recognizing that there are many different approaches that can be taken when developing and implementing health promotion initiatives (Rojas-Guyler et al., 2007). The major activities to accomplish include building relationships with community agencies, defining issues to address, planning community-based health interventions, and implementing and evaluating the health promotion intervention.

Building Relationships With Community Agencies

Good collaboration is critical to the success of community-based health promotion programs (Sogoric et al., 2005). Time needs to be spent on infrastructure development wherein the inter-agency or collaborative structure and mission are defined and decision-making processes established (Yoo et al., 2003). It takes time to develop this infrastructure, as the partners will need to consider the different imperatives under which their agencies function in order to arrive at workable processes for collaboration (Yoo et al., 2003). The work to establish infrastructure does not take place in isolation; rather, it will emerge as agency representatives define the issues to address and prioritize activities. Inevitably organizational restrictions (e.g., policy, mission) or legal imperatives under which the collaborating partners operate will be identified that must be taken into consideration in the planning process. Relationship building is ongoing throughout collaboration and should continue even after the project is completed.

Defining Issues to Address

When working with community agencies to design health promotion initiatives, it is important for the partners to agree upon the goal or end point they are working toward. Issues salient to the community can be identified in meetings with the community partners (Yoo et al., 2003). As issues are discussed it may become necessary to expand the partnership to include representatives from the target population (e.g., ethnic groups, selected health conditions, underserved communities), government officials or neighborhood representatives, and other community agencies or organizations (Sogoric et al., 2005). The partners need to consider different dimensions that influence the health and quality of life of individuals and communities (Yoo et al., 2003).

Gathering data about the community can facilitate the partners' work to identify salient issues and create goals. Community assessments should include identifying assets and resources as well as barriers and issues of concern (Collie-Akers et al., 2007). The partners should identify previous actions taken to address the issues, assess the degree of effectiveness of the previous work, discuss how the issues affect the community, and determine the nature of the work required to address the emerging issues (Sogoric et al., 2005; Yoo et al., 2003).

Inevitably more issues will be identified than can be addressed in one intervention or project. It will be necessary for the partners to prioritize the identified issues and select those that can be tackled by the community partners (Yoo et al., 2003). Prioritization can be made based on a number of criteria, including the time-sensitive nature of the issue, available resources for addressing the issue, complexity of the issue, and severity of the issue. A wise strategy for new collaborators to follow would be to select an issue that is manageable in scope, fits the available resources (both financial and non-financial), and has a good potential for success. Success with smaller projects can serve as the impetus to tackle more complex projects.

Planning a Community-Based Health Intervention

After an issue is selected and a goal defined, the partners need to create a plan of action to organize their work (Yoo et al., 2003). Members of the planning committee need to include representatives of the target community, whether it is a specific neighborhood or a selected health condition, so that the action plan can be adapted to meet the target population's needs. Sogoric et al. (2005) found that the most effective health promotion interventions were those that had been adapted based on consumers' input.

The action plan will include identified tasks to be accomplished with a timeline for task implementation (Yoo et al., 2003). Responsibility will be assigned to partners for completing the different tasks. Incorporating process evaluation in the action plan will assist the partners in refining the plan to meet changing conditions (Sogoric et al., 2005).

As the partners create and refine the action plan, they will need to determine the type and quantity of resources needed to implement the plan. Financial support is needed for some but not all of the tasks. Some resources may be provided by the partners, such as meeting space, duplication services, news items or ads in newsletters or flyers that are routinely produced by the agency, volunteers, and clerical support (Goddard, 2004). No-cost resources should also be sought, such as free advertising through public service announcements on local television and radio stations and the educational materials available from national health-based organizations. Other resources may require funding, and so a task force may be organized to develop and submit proposals to foundations or other charitable organizations seeking grants to support the project.

Implementing the Health Promotion Intervention

The action plan will guide the implementation of the intervention. Effective health promotion interventions include process and summative evaluations.

The action plan should include procedures for obtaining feedback from both the consumers and the interveners during implementation and after the intervention is completed (Yoo et al., 2003). Community partners and members of the planning committee need to use the process evaluation data to identify and correct problems during implementation. Wherever possible, the planners should identify alternate plans in anticipation of potential roadblocks (Yoo et al., 2003). Common challenges faced when implementing community-based health promotion programs include soliciting community members' participation, inadequate or incomplete assessments of community assets and barriers, maintaining intervention fidelity or consistency across intervention sessions, allocating sufficient time to carry out activities, and obtaining community data for planning and evaluating the program (Sogoric et al., 2005; Yoo et al., 2003).

Evaluating the Health Promotion Intervention

Evaluation is an ongoing activity throughout implementation of the program and should include feedback on the process, the program itself, and ideally health or quality of life outcomes. Process evaluation should provide the community partners with information to respond to situational factors that can affect the program (Sogoric et al., 2005). Informal process evaluation includes regular debriefing of the intervention facilitators by the partners (Yoo et al., 2003). Summative evaluation should include program satisfaction and measures pertaining to the selected health or health-related outcomes. In addition, the planners should evaluate achievements gained through provision of the health promotion intervention, such as increased public awareness of the health issue and changes in individual health behaviors or community health resources as a result of the collaborative efforts of the community partners (Sogoric et al., 2005).

Maintaining Collaborative Relationships

Establishing collaborative relationships with community agencies, while challenging, is well worth the CNS's investment. The CNS needs to continue investing time and effort in maintaining these relationships. As noted earlier, success in implementing health promotion projects can lead to further and potentially more comprehensive collaborations that have the potential to benefit the greater community. Having established a working relationship with community agencies, the CNS may then be able to facilitate the entrée of colleagues into community agencies to further serve the greater community. Factors that were found to be critical to successful community-based collaborative health interventions included:

- Identifying an important unmet need;
- Having people with the necessary skills, expertise, and commitment to see the project through to completion;
- Paying careful attention to the planning process;
- Good collaboration between the partners;
- Having an inclusive leadership style; and
- Maintaining a clear focus on the targeted consumers of the program. (Sogoric et al., 2005)

16.1 Reaching Out to Community Agencies: Getting Started

1. Identify community agencies
   - Agencies that provide health care services or resources:
     - Hospitals
     - Clinics
     - Health department
     - Hospice
     - Medical supply vendors
     - Emergency medical services
     - Morgue
     - Funeral/mortuary vendors
   - Organizations/groups with primary focus on health care:
     - Professional associations
     - Support groups
     - School nurses
     - Parish nurses
   - Other community agencies:
     - Churches, synagogues, temples
     - Schools, colleges, universities
     - Parks & leisure programs
     - Library
     - Exercise facilities
     - Transportation vendors
2. Contact community agencies
   - Volunteer services, general
   - Volunteer to serve on specific project
   - Search for collaborative projects
   - Propose collaborative projects
3. Working with community agencies
   - Building relationships
   - Defining issues to address
   - Planning a community-based health intervention
   - Implementing the interventions
   - Evaluation: process, product, outcome
4. Maintaining collaborative relationships
   - Invest time to maintain relationships
   - Facilitate entrée of colleagues into organization

In summary, reaching out to community agencies is a vital option for building a community's capacity to effectively improve the health of the community. Given the dwindling resources available to community agencies, local governments, and health care institutions, the CNS can build collaborative relationships designed to fill community health needs. Table 16.1 summarizes the points made in this chapter.

References

Collie-Akers, V. L., Fawcett, S. B., Schultz, J. A., Carson, V., Cyprus, J., & Pierle, J. E. (2007). Analyzing a community-based coalition's efforts to reduce health disparities and the risk for chronic disease in Kansas City, Missouri. *Preventing Chronic Disease, 4*(3). Retrieved July 23, 2007, from http://www.cdc.gov/pcd/issues/2007/jul/06_0101.htm

Goddard, T. (2004). Can corporate sector philanthropy be included in a new vision for community health programs? *Australian Occupational Therapy Journal, 51*, 106–109.

National Association of Clinical Nurse Specialists (NACNS)—Statement Revision Task Force. (2004). *Statement on clinical nurse specialist practice and education* (2nd ed.). Harrisburg, PA: Author.

National Center for Health Statistics. (2006). *Health, United States, 2006, with chartbook on trends in the health of Americans.* Hyattsville, MD: Author.

Rojas-Guyler, L., Murnan, J., & Cottrell, R. R. (2007). Networking for career-long success: A powerful strategy for health education professionals. *Health Promotion Practice, 8*, 229–233.

Sogoric, S., Middleton, J., Lang, S., Ivankovic, D., & Kern, J. (2005). A naturalistic inquiry on the impact of interventions aiming to improve health and the quality of life in the community. *Social Science & Medicine, 60*, 153–164.

Yoo, S., Shada, R. E., Goodman, R. M., Weed, N. E., Lempa, M. L., & Mbondo, M. (2003). Collaborative community empowerment: An illustration of a six-step process. *Health Promotion Practice, 4*, 1–10.

Young, T. K. (2005). *Population health: Concepts and methods* (2nd ed.). New York: Oxford University Press.

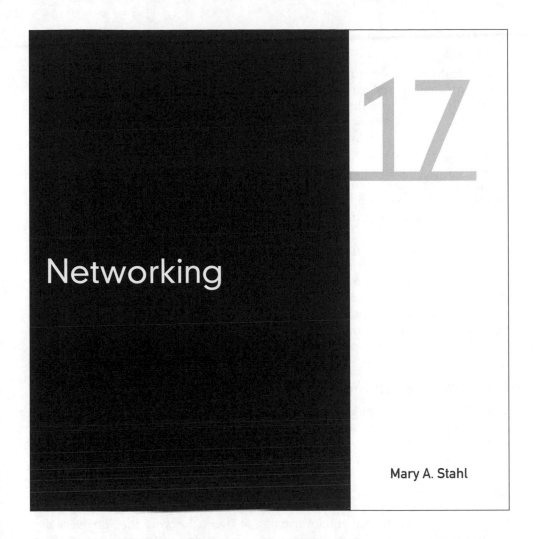

Networking

Mary A. Stahl

Networking is a valuable activity in any profession. The clinical nurse specialist (CNS) will find that networking can expedite and add value to contributions in the workplace, stimulate new ideas and approaches to problems, provide opportunities for professional skill development and awareness of career opportunities, and increase personal satisfaction. This chapter will describe networking on a variety of levels, starting within the employment setting, then in the local community, and finally on a broader scale. A variety of examples will be identified to provide ideas on how to access these networks and the types of opportunities they will provide.

What is networking? According to the organization Women Into the Network, networking is simply "connecting with people of like interests and uncovering opportunities" (n.d., ¶ 1). Networking is forming relationships with other people to learn and grow from the reciprocal exchange of ideas, advice, and experiences (Scott, 2007). While communicating with people we know is an everyday activity, the purposeful approach of establishing contacts for networking may feel uncomfortable to some. The benefits, however, are well worth the effort.

Basically you are getting to know people and they are getting to know you. Be open, friendly, and an astute listener. Have a question in mind as an ice-breaker that relates to the situation where you are meeting others, and show a genuine interest to learn about them. If you are new to a work setting, the question "What brought you to work here?" will generally get people talking and may give you useful information about your employer. Asking others about their work—or if outside your work setting, their thoughts on a speaker or conference you are both attending—may be an easy way to open a conversation. Be comfortable talking about yourself both professionally and personally.

If there is an opportunity to provide information or a resource that is of interest to the other person, do so as long as this doesn't disclose information that is confidential to your employer. Some employers consider protocols, order sets, and the like to be proprietary and will not want you sharing with organizations that they consider to be competitors. Sharing resources when possible and sharing experiences and ideas help form a positive impression that will aid in developing at least a contact or perhaps a relationship. To dispel a misconception from the business community, the goal is the relationship, not identifying what the other person can do for you.

Networking Within Your Hospital or System

When starting a new position, some initial contacts, such as your immediate supervisor or the person assigned to help with orientation to the institution and role, will be identified for you. Others will become apparent in your clinical area, such as the clinical and formal leaders and the multidisciplinary team members. Relationships with the physicians most frequently encountered in your practice area are well worth cultivating so that practice issues and change projects will be easier to negotiate when they arise. The nursing staff will help you understand the processes, both formal and informal, that frame the work they do every day. Their insights will help you understand what is working and what is not working, and will identify the work-arounds that occur on a routine basis. This will help you understand where to focus your efforts to make the most meaningful contributions to patient safety, clinical excellence, and unit culture. Key relationships to develop will include the CNSs and other advanced practice nurses (APNs) within the hospital and system. They will be invaluable in helping you understand the ways in which APNs have had impact in the organization, and will have insight into the formal and informal approval processes. If your hospital is part of a health care system, developing relationships in other system entities can be valuable, particularly in the clinical areas most similar to your practice.

Be alert to opportunities to develop relationships throughout the organization. Participation in various projects and workgroups may bring contact with administrators, a quality analyst, the person who negotiates insurance payor contracts, or the Risk Management department, among others. These are unique opportunities to network, not only putting a face with a name, but creating an impression so when you reach out with a question or request the person is likely to remember you.

The relationships developed within your work environment will be crucial in day-to-day activities and in your ability to create change. These individuals can contribute different perspectives to help fully analyze an issue and evaluate potential solutions. They will include key leaders whose support will move projects forward and can provide insight to address barriers. Some will be able to provide a broader view of the organization and other initiatives that are occurring, which will be valuable information as you anticipate challenges and opportunities for your practice area and for your involvement at the institutional or system level.

Networking Within Your Local Community

Developing relationships beyond your institution in your local community also brings value. Seek groups with like interests, such as CNS or APN groups, local chapters of national clinical specialty groups, or Sigma Theta Tau chapters (see Chapter 15, "Becoming Involved With Professional Organizations"). Individuals you meet through these groups will have interests in common with you. Find opportunities to make connections within local academic institutions. Local educational programs provide the opportunity to meet colleagues from other hospitals in your area. Become active in voluntary health agencies, volunteering your time and expertise. Even participation in community or civic groups may yield networking chances; take the opportunity to get to know people through your faith organization, children's school, or at the dog park or community events.

These networking opportunities may provide an expanded view of your institution within the community. If you are considering changing positions, you may learn of job opportunities or have the chance to learn about other employers in ways that do not come through in an interview. Viewpoints from outside your organization may help bring new perspectives on issues you are addressing or new ideas for solutions. You may find mentors or the opportunity to collaborate on projects that benefit multiple hospitals, such as a stroke education consortium, multi-site research, or performance improvement project (Kleinpell & Hravnak, 2005). If you are working with a program that reaches into the community for health screening and promotion or education, contacts within community organizations may facilitate access to target populations or help refine your approach.

Networking on a Broader Scale

With the skills and confidence you have developed through networking in your local area, you are now ready to expand your network to a national or even international level. Attending a national conference provides numerous opportunities to network: in the registration line, lunch line, or as you wait for a session to begin. Take advantage of social opportunities and events that are created for just this purpose. Easy icebreakers may be "Where do you work?" or a comment on one of the speakers or sessions you have enjoyed. Some conferences recruit attendees to introduce speakers. This can be an opportunity to meet someone you admire or who has done work on a topic in which you are interested. Professional organizations, special interest groups, and journals not only provide practice and professional resources, but contact information for authors and leaders can often be obtained through their Web sites. These create networking opportunities when their expertise relates to an area of your interest. Your own publications in newsletters and journals may draw contacts, not only with editors and guest editors but also with those who read your work.

Electronic mailing lists, commonly called Listservs, are a convenient way to reach out to a large number of people who are interested in a given topic area. One of the many electronic mailing lists you may find of value to you is the CNS Listserv, which can be joined by sending a blank e-mail to cns-listserv-on@mail-list.com from the e-mail account where you wish to receive messages. An electronic mailing list is a network of people who share questions, answers, examples from their practice, and their thoughts about various topics. Posts from members are received as e-mail to which you can choose to respond if you have something to contribute. You can post your own questions as well, and gain thoughts, support, and sometimes examples of tools or protocols from a wide network of colleagues, sometimes from all over the world. On subscribing to an electronic mailing list you will be notified of communication norms and you will start by introducing yourself to the group. You will get to know many of the electronic mailing list members from their frequent posts and will find opportunities to communicate with them beyond the electronic mailing list if you choose. Messages posted to the group are usually archived by the list software. Using the information in the e-mail welcome message, you can access these archives in case you need to refresh your memory of the information that has been shared. Archives are organized by threads, which are the subject lines in e-mail messages (Thede, 2007).

There are a variety of Internet approaches to networking that have been effective in other industries and may be of value to the CNS. Chat rooms may help you make contact with others who share your interests. These are Internet sites that resemble live group discussions conducted by text or in some cases Web cam. Chat rooms are often organized around a broad topic focus. Bulletin boards are Web sites where members post discussion threads and others post comments. Rather than receiving each post by e-mail, as you would on an electronic mailing list, you visit the Web site on a regular basis to see what others have written and to post your messages. Some chat rooms and bulletin boards require you to become a member to access the messages. Others are in the public domain and are accessible to all. Particularly in the public domain, remember safety rules such as using a screen name and making sure you do not give out personal information that could be used to locate you.

Blogs are longer narrative postings created by an individual. These may relate the individual's experiences, or thoughts and opinions around a topic. Bloggers commonly post these monologs on a regular basis, and readers have the opportunity to post their comments and views in response. Blogs may create a networking opportunity if you find a blogger you admire. You can leave comments about their blogs on a regular basis, and they will learn to recognize those who leave thoughtful comments. Bloggers like to help people in their blog community (Trunk, n.d., ¶ 26), so if you have a request and they recognize you from your comments, you have made a useful contact.

Another Internet networking opportunity may be social networks. Some, such as Facebook, primarily provide a way to stay connected with a group of people you already know. Others target business networking or create a method for those who are looking for jobs to list a professional profile (Fox, 2007; Kadlec, 2007). In the business community there is a trend for employers or recruiters to seek potential employees through these social networks, so there is the potential that in the future this might become a job search strategy in health care.

Networking With Industry

The CNS often has many opportunities to work with representatives from industry. Sales representatives and clinical experts from a variety of pharmaceutical, technology, and medical product companies seek out the CNS either to promote their products or to provide educational support for safe, appropriate use of their products. While this is a valuable resource, do not ignore the additional networking opportunities these contacts provide. There are multiple opportunities here, ranging from influencing product development and participating in pre- or post-market research, to working as an educational consultant, or even potential employment. These representatives can also be tapped to exhibit at and financially support educational programs or conferences you may be coordinating. If you are seeking contacts in industry, you can contact them through Internet sites or meet them in the exhibit hall at professional conferences.

Benefits of Networking

The benefits of networking will be realized in day-to-day work as a CNS, through skill development, professional opportunities, career mobility, and personal satisfaction. While the relationships you develop within your organization will facilitate your involvement in the right projects and the success of your initiatives, the connections developed outside provide an opportunity to compare practices across a wide range of settings. The creative strategies, barriers and how to address them, and outcomes from practice changes accomplished by others can provide depth to your planning and increase your successes. At the very least you will gain valuable information to enrich your practice and bring new ideas to your workplace (Nicholl & Tracey, 2007).

Collaboration and mentoring opportunities result from networking. You can find opportunities to hone presentation skills or develop competencies in publishing or editorial work. A mentor may help you expand your research skills or provide opportunities for collaborative research. Communication with leaders and others with diverse perspectives and participation in dialogue about professional trends and national issues will further develop your perspective and the depth of your thinking. Connections can lead to involvement and leadership roles in community activities and professional organizations, and involvement in legislative or regulatory activities. You can find opportunities to serve as a mentor yourself, sharing your expertise with others.

The relationships you build may result in role expansion with joint appointment as clinical or academic faculty. Employment and entrepreneurial opportunities may come your way. If you are interested in relocating to another city, connections you make can give you a personal insight into that community or hospital and local support as you are getting established in your new community.

Once you have established solid relationships, there is even the opportunity to actively engage selected individuals in projects of your own. You might seek individuals from your network to contribute to a journal issue for which you are serving as guest editor, or as speakers at a conference you are working to organize. Rich, Hart, Barrett, Marks, and Ruderman (1995) describe a group of CNSs who formed a peer consultation group. The purpose of the group was to continue to learn together and support one another in professional development. Typical activities included group consultation about clinical situations and group mentoring around professional skill development, such as presentation skills. Ward (2006) describes creating a network focused on developing new approaches to shared problems. He purposefully recruited a cadre of people who would engage in learning activities, discussion, and group projects as a way to challenge themselves to develop new approaches to their work. Ward assigned specific literature, posed questions, and assigned individual and group tasks for the purpose of stimulating thought and creativity within his group. Experimentation was encouraged. The goal was to develop a network of innovative thought leaders. Perhaps one of these examples triggers your own ideas of how you might engage selected members of your network to achieve shared goals.

Networking not only opens doors, it helps you develop so you can confidently step through those doors and contribute in a multitude of ways to the growth of the profession. The resulting experiences will enrich your career in countless ways.

References

Fox, V. (2007). Searching for people in all the new social places. *Information Today, 24*(8), 25.

Kadlec, D. (2007). You oughta be in Facebook. *Money, 36*(10), 44.

Kleinpell, R. M., & Hravnak, M. M. (2005). Strategies for success in the acute care nurse practitioner role. *Critical Care Nursing Clinics of North America, 17,* 177–181.

Nicholl, H., & Tracey, C. (2007). Networking for nurses. *Nursing Management, 13*(9), 26–29.

Rich, B. W., Hart, B., Barrett, A., Marks, G., & Ruderman, S. (1995). Peer consultation: A look at process. *Clinical Nurse Specialist, 9*(3), 181–185.

Scott, D. E. (2007). Networking Series Part I: Networking fundamentals for nurses. *Wyoming Nurse* (Sept., Oct., Nov.), 12.

Thede, L. Q. (2007). Networking via e-mail. *CIN: Computers, Informatics, Nursing* (Sept.–Oct.), 251–253.

Trunk, P. (n.d.). Networking for people who hate networking. Retrieved February 9, 2008, from http://finance.yahoo.com/expert/article/careerist/27020

Ward, D. (2006). Project blue lynx: An innovative approach to mentoring and networking. *Defense AT&L* (July–August), 34–37.

Women Into the Network. (n.d.). What is networking and how can it be of benefit to my business? Retrieved February 9, 2008, from http://www.womenintothenetwork.co.uk/page/howtonetwork.cfm

VI

Professional Recognition

18

Obtaining Certification: Considering the Options

Melanie Duffy

You've come a long way from an undergraduate in a nursing program to a graduate student in a clinical nurse specialist (CNS) program. You've negotiated a job, perhaps wrote your own job description, and figured out where you fit into the organization. Many projects have come your way. New responsibilities and expectations have been placed upon you by others. Now you're probably thinking, "What's next?" Well, the next step in your professional growth and development is certification. Yes, you've thought about it. You even have colleagues who are certified. But now the time has come for you to take the next logical step in your professional career as an advanced practice nurse (APN).

Meanings of Certification

Certification has several meanings depending on the context of the conversation. Certification is not a legal term, however. Professional licensure is a legal term because it is a requirement to practice nursing. Certification, on the other hand, is voluntary. A specific employer may require certification as a condition of employment, but it is not a legal requirement. Certification may have a different meaning depending on the state in which you practice. For example, in Pennsylvania, certification means that you have been approved by the State Board of Nursing (SBN) to practice as an APN. Nurse practitioners are certified to practice in the state, but the term connotes approval by the SBN.

Certification carries another meaning. Certification implies protection of the public. The certified CNS has gone above and beyond the basic requirements needed to practice as an APN. The CNS has experience (perhaps years) and advanced knowledge in a specialty area. The CNS has practiced in that specialty and kept abreast of new technologies and treatment modalities. And finally, the CNS has successfully passed a certification examination. Today's health care consumer is aware of what is involved in the certification process and has added confidence in the certified nurse providing care.

Certification and Professional Organizations

Certification is defined by the American Board of Nursing Specialties (ABNS, 2005) as the formal recognition of specialized knowledge, skills, and experience demonstrated by the achievement of standards identified by a nursing specialty to promote optimal health outcomes. ABNS, a nonprofit organization, accredits specialty nursing certification examination programs. ABNS maintains standards to which certifying nursing organizations adhere. The mission of ABNS is to promote the value of specialty nursing certification. The public recognizes quality nursing care according to the standard of specialty certification (ABNS, 2005).

Many nursing organizations have certification options at different levels. Certification may be available for nurses with specialized practice knowledge and skill, such as in oncology, critical care, or rehabilitation. Nurses are not required to have advanced education at the basic or generalist level of specialty-focused certification. Nurses with associate or bachelor degrees may be eligible for certification. Advanced level certification may be available in the same specialty for nurses with graduate preparation in areas such as oncology CNS or critical care CNS. Some certifying bodies have only one certification option (for the nurse practicing with a basic knowledge of the specialty), while others offer both basic and advanced.

The American Association of Critical Care Nurses Certification Corporation (AACN cert. corp.) has several certification options available for nurses practicing at both basic and advanced levels. For example, AACN cert. corp. has basic level certification in the specialty areas of critical care, progressive care, cardiac medicine, and cardiac surgery. AACN cert. corp. has a certification examination available at the advanced level for the CNS providing care to the adult, critically ill population (American Association of Critical Care Nurses [AACN], 2006a).

The American Nurses Credentialing Center, an arm of the American Nurses Association, also has several specialty certifications for the APN. For example, certification is available for CNSs in adult health, pediatrics, and community health (American Nurses Credentialing Center, 2008). The Oncology Nursing Certification Corporation (2008) also has an advanced level certification for the CNS—advanced oncology clinical nurse specialist (AOCNS).

The National Association of Clinical Nurse Specialists (NACNS, 2005) supports certification at the advanced practice level. The CNS was the first advanced practice nurse to be recognized to have a unique body of knowledge and

18.1 CNS Certification Options

Organization	Title	Credential	Web Site
American Nurses Credentialing Center	Adult Health CNS-Board Certified	ACNS-BC	http://www.nurse credentialing.org/cert
	Gerontological CNS-Board Certified	GCNS-BC	
	Home Health CNS-Board Certified	HHCNS-BC	
	Pediatric CNS-Board Certified	PCNS-BC	
	Psychiatric Mental Health CNS-Board Certified (appropriate for Child/Adolescent and Adult populations)	PMHCNS-BC	
AACN Certification Corporation	Critical Care CNS (appropriate for Adult, Neonatal, and Pediatric populations)	CCNS	http://www.certcorp.org
Oncology Nursing Certification Corporation	Advanced Oncology CNS	AOCNS	http://www.oncc.org

competencies based on education at the graduate level (Mick & Ackerman, 2002). Verification of advanced knowledge in a specialty area can be accomplished via advanced education at the master's or doctoral level. Most certification options use psychometric examinations to measure knowledge; however, other scientifically sound and legally defensible methods, such as a portfolio, are possible and are being explored for further application (NACNS, 2005). Table 18.1 lists a few examples of currently available CNS certification options.

One problem, as you probably have already surmised, is that there are numerous advanced practice specialties but few certification options for verifying CNS specialty knowledge, but more about that later.

Rationale for Certification

Why should you become certified? After all, becoming certified means you'd likely have to take a *test* and *pass* it!! Well, there is a little bit more to it than just studying for and passing a test. First of all, talk to your colleagues and ask why they pursued certification. Several reasons in support of certification will be evident. First, certification is validation of your knowledge by a professional body.

Yes, you will probably have to study to be successful with the test, but your advanced knowledge is already there. You just have to brush up on a few things.

Second, professional certification demonstrates to the public that the holder of a certification credential has demonstrated knowledge of practice standards in a specialty area. Boards of nursing often use professional certification as a proxy for knowledge in a specialty and issue a state certificate to practice as an APN/CNS based on professional certification. Certification, such as Critical Care Clinical Nurse Specialist (CCNS), is a professional credential. Protection of the public is the state's issue specifically. A state may ask for and/or accept the professional credential as part of a procedure to protect the public. Advanced level certification signals competence, advanced abilities, and confidence to the consumer.

Third, your employer benefits from your certification. A CNS who obtains professional certification contributes to the overall reputation of the health care setting in which he/she practices. The consumer recognizes that the health care setting invests in an APN who has greater accountability for actions and ensures delivery of evidence-based, quality care. Liability rates for the employee/employer may decrease (AACN, 2006b).

Fourth, you will have a reputation as a certified CNS. Certification builds self-confidence about knowledge and expertise, and gives you the satisfaction of having achieved a prestigious personal goal. Your accomplishment will serve to inspire colleagues to also seek certification. Perhaps you will be the one giving advice to others who wish to pursue certification. Last, some employers provide financial support for certification or incentives to achieve and maintain certification. Check to see if your employer offers financial support for a review course and/or reimbursement for costs incurred to take the exam. Ask about a financial bonus/salary adjustment for successful completion of the exam or if certification will be positively reflected in your annual performance review and/or merit-based salary increase.

The Decision Is Made: Test-Taking Skills

You finally made the decision to take the plunge! You invested in a review book with sample questions in your specialty. You reviewed the test blueprint, available on most nursing organization Web sites. Perhaps you became part of a study group so you wouldn't have to embark on the project alone. Maybe you made flash cards with bits and pieces of information that were difficult for you to grasp. Audiotapes were also a good investment since you have a long commute to work and sit in traffic.

How will you actually prepare for the test? Dennison offers some helpful hints on how to prepare to take the test and be successful (Dennison & Rollant, 2002).

First, use practice questions. Ask why you missed the question if you chose the incorrect answer. Read the question thoroughly. Highlight key points as you read the question. Answer the question after you read the stem without looking at the options. Read all options as well as the stem. Eliminate clearly incorrect options. Eliminate similar options that say the same thing. Choose the answer that matches the question in scope. If the question is general, give a general answer; if the question is specific, give a specific answer.

Second, do not assume information that is not given. All important information is included in the stem. Included information is probably important.

Third, answer the easy questions first. Return to the difficult questions later. Do not leave any questions blank.

Select an answer according to clinical priority. Start with the most life-threatening problems. Think airway, breathing, and circulation! Next consider the seriousness of a complication if interventions are missed. Think long-term consequences and disability. Next, consider pain and comfort. Acute pain is a priority unless a life-threatening situation is present. Actual problems always take precedence over potential problems. Use the nursing process to determine next steps if the question asks what to do next in a situation. Use Maslow's hierarchy of needs to determine the initial need if the question asks what a patient needs. Focus on patient safety if the patient doesn't have an urgent physiologic need. Choose actions to check the patient first and the equipment second. Look at the big picture and the organ systems affected. The pulmonary and cardiovascular systems are the priority in life-threatening situations.

Avoid outright guessing. If you are not sure, first try to eliminate any choices that are obviously or most likely incorrect. Make your best choice from the remaining options.

Maintaining concentration is also a test-taking skill. Rephrase a question rather than rereading the same question over and over. Write down normal lab values or formulas on scrap paper before you answer the first question. Read the answers in reverse order—option d to option a. Take some slow, deep breaths to refocus and regroup. Or you may find a quick trip to the restroom will facilitate renewed thinking capabilities.

Changing answers—should you or shouldn't you? Be aware of your specific pattern of errors. If you miss questions because you don't read them thoroughly, then of course change the answers. But if you miss questions even though you read them thoroughly, don't change the initial answers.

Budget your time. Generally certification exams provide sufficient time to complete the task. Proceed quickly and carefully through the questions, but don't spend too much time on any one question. You can always come back to it.

Lastly, don't cram the night before the exam. Go to bed at a reasonable time. Wear comfortable, layered clothes the day of the exam. Eat a light, healthy meal. Avoid the Danish or donut. Eat something with protein and a little fat to carry you through to the end of the task. Perhaps an egg sandwich or an apple with a little peanut butter. And think positively!

No Certification Available? Now What?

Numerous advanced practice specialties exist, but few certification options are available. Why doesn't every specialty have a certification option? Well, for one reason, it is cost-prohibitive. To produce a psychometrically sound and legally defensible examination to validate knowledge costs hundreds of thousands of dollars. Most nursing organizations are relatively small, have few members, and can't afford the financial commitment. Grants and donations may be options for examination development but may not be able to support continued maintenance. Examinations are constructed using expert panels that determine the content and write the individual test items. This process is required for initial test development and ongoing test updates. Overall, the ongoing process is very expensive. The expense of developing and offering the certification exam will not be recoverable for small specialty practice groups for which the test takers pool is limited.

So what's the alternative? One option is to successfully complete specialty certification at the basic knowledge level if an advanced version is not available. You still will have demonstrated expertise in a specialty, will be a role model for your colleagues and staff nurses, will have contributed to your institution's reputation, and will have gained financially.

A second option is to demonstrate your knowledge and expertise through submission of a portfolio. A portfolio is a compendium document that reflects practice competencies and may include examples of specific patient cases; projects developed, implemented, and completed; products, equipment, actions of medications, and treatment modalities evaluated; research and evidence-based projects completed; continuing education activities; podium/poster presentations at local, regional, national, and international conferences and professional meetings; and nurses mentored. Collectively, the examples in the portfolio provide a comprehensive and in-depth reflection of an individual's CNS practice.

Summary

Certification is the next logical step in your professional career as a CNS. Do it now. Don't put it off. There's no time like the present. Join your certified colleagues as one with a validated knowledge base and demonstrated expertise in a specialty. Become accountable and responsible for your actions above a basic level. The certification designation will only add to your exemplary career as a CNS.

References

American Association of Critical Care Nurses. (2006a). *AACN certification corporation fact sheet*. Retrieved September 7, 2007, from http://www.certcorp.org

American Association of Critical Care Nurses. (2006b). *Nurse certification benefits patients, employers and nurses*. Retrieved September 7, 2007, from http://www.certcorp.org

American Board of Nursing Specialties. (2005). *A position statement on the value of specialty nursing certification*. Retrieved September 7, 2007, from http://www.nursingcertification.org

American Nurses Credentialing Center. (2008). Retrieved September 7, 2007, from http://www.ancc.org

Dennison, R., & Rollant, P. (2002). *Testtaking techniques: Review and resource manual*. Washington, DC: Institute for Research, Education, and Consultation at the American Nurses Credentialing Center.

Mick, D. J., & Ackerman, M. H. (2002). Deconstructing the myth of the advanced practice blended role: Support for role divergence. *Heart and Lung, 31*(6), 393–398.

National Association of Clinical Nurse Specialists (NACNS). (2005). *White paper on certification of clinical nurse specialists*. Retrieved September 7, 2007, from http://www.nacns.org

Oncology Nursing Society. (2008). Retrieved February 11, 2008, from http://www.ons.org

19

Navigating the Privileging and Credentialing Process

Susan Sendelbach

Credentialing and privileging are mandated by the Joint Commission (JC) to protect patients to ensure that professionals within the institution are competent and practicing within their scopes of practice (Magdic, Hravnak, & McCartney, 2005). Historically, only physicians were credentialed and privileged. However, in 1983 JC established new regulations that allowed non-physician providers on medical staff as allied health professionals (Stanley, 2005). This change allowed the credentialing and privileging of advanced practice registered nurses (APRNs), including clinical nurse specialists (CNSs). The credentialing and privileging process is important to CNSs because it supports appropriate peer review of competency and qualifications for the practice roles, enables third-party reimbursement, and promotes self-regulation and quality of patient care (Finch-Guthrie, 2006). Each hospital has the responsibility of ensuring that APRNs who practice within their institution are credentialed, privileged, and re-privileged through the medical staff process or a procedure that is equivalent (Joint Commission, 2009). Although credentialing and privileging are two different processes, they are usually done in parallel.

What Is Credentialing?

The American Nurses Association (ANA) defines credentialing as "the process of assessing and validating the qualifications of a licensed independent practitioner to provide patient care services based on an evaluation of the individual's licensure, training, experience, current competence, and the ability to perform the requested privileges" (American Nurses Association [ANA], 2006). This process is used by health care organizations; it involves obtaining and verifying a CNS's licensure, clinical experience, and preparation in a specialty practice (Joint Commission, 2009; Klein, 2003). Verification of education and relevant training should be obtained from primary sources including, for example, letters from schools documenting satisfactory completion of program requirement or degree conferred (Joint Commission, 2009). The credentialing process can be conducted by the hospital, through the human resource department or department of medical affairs, or delegated to a credential verification organization (CVO) as specified in the medical staff bylaws of the institution, based on the recommendations of the medical staff, and as approved by the governing body (Joint Commission, 2009; Kamajian, Mitchell, & Fruth, 1999). The overall goal of verifying credentials is to ensure that the applicant's qualifications are consistent with the position's responsibilities and that the applicant is appropriately prepared to perform the duties implied by the credential (Hamric, Spross, & Hanson, 2005).

What Is Privileging?

Privileging is the "authorization granted by the governing body of a healthcare facility, agency, or organization to provide specific patient care service within well-defined limits, based on qualifications reviewed in the credentials process" (ANA, 2006). The process includes developing and approving a procedure list; processing the application; evaluating applicant-specific information; submitting recommendations to the governing body for applicant-specific delineated privileges; notifying the applicant and relevant personnel of the privileging decision; and monitoring the use of privileges and quality of care issues (Joint Commission, 2009). The privileges that a CNS requests will differ by state, since all CNSs practice within the scope of practice as defined in the individual state's Nurse Practice Act. The state in which the CNS practices determines the limits and privileges of the CNS license (Finch-Guthrie, 2006; Kamajian et al., 1999). Thus, the individual state's scope of practice for the CNS will determine which patients the CNS can see and treat; what circumstance or guidance a CNS will need to provide care; and the minimum level of CNS competency (Finch-Guthrie, 2006). For example, a CNS may need to have a collaborative agreement with a physician to be able to prescribe medications. This would be defined by the state's scope of practice.

Joint Commission (2009) mandates that the applicant's ability to perform requested privileges be evaluated. This includes documentation that the applicant has no health problems that could affect his or her practice; JC recommends this be confirmed (Joint Commission, 2009). In addition, when applying for privileges, the National Practitioner Data Bank (NPDB) is queried to potentially discover proceedings and reports against an applicant. The NPDB, established in 1986 and implemented in 1990, receives, stores, and disseminates information on malpractice payments and disciplinary sanctions against health care practitioners (Waters, Warnecke, Parsons, Almagor, & Budetti, 2006).

As a part of the privileging process, peer recommendation is required and includes written information about the applicant's clinical knowledge; technical and clinical skills; clinical judgment; interpersonal skills; communication skills; and professionalism (Joint Commission, 2009). An evaluation of the requested information is conducted before recommending approval of privileges. The hospital must have a process to determine if there is sufficient clinical performance to make a decision to grant, limit, or deny the privilege requested by the applicant. A period of focused professional practice evaluation is required for all initially requested privileges, is defined by the organized medical staff, and can include activities such as chart review and monitoring clinical practice patterns. Joint Commission (2009) also requires that the re-privileging process take place at least every two years.

Special considerations of the credentialing and privileging process include an expedited process that may be used for an initial appointment; temporary privileges that allow for temporary clinical privileges for a limited time period; disaster privileges that will allow privileges to volunteers eligible to be licensed independent practitioners; and a process for the practice of telemedicine (Joint Commission, 2009).

The Credentialing and Privileging Process

ANA recommends the nursing peer review within the credentialing and privileging process be conducted by other APRNs and suggests one of two models (ANA, 2006). The first is the Nursing Model, in which the nursing peer review committee reviews and recommends to the chief nursing officer (CNO), who then reviews and credentials the APRN. The second is the Collaborative Model, in which the nursing peer review committee initially reviews and approves the APRN credentialing application, consistent with the institution's policy, and final approval is granted by the institution's Credentialing Committee. Regardless of the model chosen, it is important that APRNs be a part of the process in order to support the principle of self-regulation. ANA (2006) views the credentialing and privileging of APRNs, including CNSs, as critical processes that help support the full scope of practice for the APRN. In addition, the Magnet Standards support the autonomous practice of nurses, including APRNs. One source of evidence used to examine an institution is "the process by which advanced practice nurses are credentialed, privileged, and evaluated" (American Nurses Credentialing Center [ANCC], 2005, p. 55). The CNO must also submit documentation of his or her participation (or designee) in the privileging process for advanced practice nurses (ANCC, 2005). Clearly the credentialing and privileging of APRNs is becoming the standard, as opposed to the exception.

In summary, although the credentialing and privileging process may seem to be arduous, it is vital to ensure patient quality of care. Additionally, the process promotes the full scope of practice for APRNs and provides for self-regulation of CNSs and CNS practice.

References

American Nurses Association. (2006, October 11). *Credentialing and privileging of advanced practice registered nurses.* Retrieved January 21, 2008, from http://www.nursingworld.org/MainMenuCategories/HealthcareandPolicyIssues/ANAPositionStatements/practice.aspx

American Nurses Credentialing Center. (2005). *The Magnet recognition program.* Silver Spring, MD: Author.

Finch-Guthrie, P. L. (2006). *Credentialing and privileging: Who? What? Why? Wherefore?* Unpublished manuscript.

Hamric, A. B., Spross, J. A., & Hanson, C. M. (2005). *Advanced practice nursing: An integrative approach* (3rd ed.). Philadelphia, PA: Elsevier.

Joint Commission. (2009, January). *Comprehensive accreditation manual.* Oakbrook Terrace, IL: Author.

Kamajian, M. F., Mitchell, S. A., & Fruth, R. A. (1999). Credentialing and privileging of advanced practice nurses. *AACN Clinical Issues: Advanced Practice in Acute & Critical Care, 10*(3), 316–336.

Klein, C. A. (2003). Legal file. The scoop on credentialing. *Nurse Practitioner, 28*(12), 54.

Magdic, K. S., Hravnak, M., & McCartney, S. (2005). Credentialing for nurse practitioners: An update. *AACN Clinical Issues: Advanced Practice in Acute & Critical Care, 16*(1), 16–22.

Stanley, J. (Ed.). (2005). *Advanced practice nursing: Emphasizing common roles* (2nd ed.). Philadelphia: F. A. Davis.

Waters, T. M., Warnecke, R. B., Parsons, J., Almagor, O., & Budetti, P. P. (2006). The role of the national practitioner data bank in the credentialing process. *American Journal of Medical Quality, 21*(1), 30–39.

20

Qualifying for Reimbursement

Susan Dresser

Clinical nurse specialists (CNSs) are continually challenged to demonstrate their value by communicating their impact on clinical outcomes, cost savings, and quality improvement. Generating revenue by billing for professional services provided is a relatively new and challenging opportunity for CNSs to demonstrate monetary value. This is a challenge for which most CNSs initially feel unprepared. Findings from a recent study of NACNS (National Association of Clinical Nurse Specialists) members by Zuzelo, Fallon, Lang, and Mount (2004) revealed that while CNSs were generally aware of Medicare structures and processes, many had basic knowledge deficits. Additionally, many lacked an understanding of federal regulations recognizing CNSs as advanced practice nurses (APNs) who could become Medicare providers and bill for services. Their findings suggested that some CNS graduate programs need to incorporate content pertaining to reimbursement methodologies. Navigating the complex, confusing, and always-changing system of rules and regulations inherent in the reimbursement arena can be overwhelming and frustrating, even for the experienced CNS. This chapter will provide an introductory overview of the coding and reimbursement processes and some insights from my own personal experience as one of the first CNSs in my state to achieve Medicare provider privileges. A brief history of the legislation that legitimized our current practice will be included.

Background of Reimbursement Legislation

The Omnibus Budget Reconciliation Act of 1989 first gave APNs the opportunity for reimbursement, although it was restricted to those practicing in skilled nursing facilities and areas designated as rural (Richmond, Thompson, & Sullivan-Marx, 2000). Several years later President Bill Clinton signed into law the historic Balanced Budget Act of 1997. This landmark legislation signified an historic victory for APNs by increasing and expanding our reimbursement opportunities. With the passage of this law, CNSs were able for the first time in history to be reimbursed by Medicare directly, regardless of geographic location or practice site. Prior to this law, direct Medicare reimbursement for APN services was limited to those services that were regarded as "physician" services and were provided in specifically defined rural areas. CNSs who provided care to Medicare patients in non-rural areas could receive reimbursement only by an indirect means known as "incident to" payments. These services had to be billed under a physician's Medicare number. The CNS had to be an employee of the physician and the reimbursement went to the physician (Abood & Keepnews, 2002).

The Balanced Budget Act expanded the definition of physicians' services to include CNSs who provide:

> services which would be physicians' services if furnished by a physician . . . and which are performed by a CNS or a NP . . . working in collaboration with a physician . . . which the nurse is legally authorized to perform by the State in which the services are performed, and such services and supplies furnished as an incident to such services as would be covered. . . . if furnished incident to a physician's professional services, but only if no facility or other provider charges or is paid any amounts with respect to the furnishing of such services. (Balanced Budget Act, 1997)

In other words, the Balanced Budget Act of 1997 authorized the Medicare program to directly reimburse CNSs when they perform what are considered to be physician services. As a result of this law, CNSs became eligible to submit claims and secure direct reimbursement from Medicare at 85% of the current physician fee or 80% of the actual charge (Balanced Budget Act, 1997). The passage of this law provided new financial opportunities for CNSs to be recognized as key health care providers, and as such, the act requires that they develop a basic understanding of reimbursement rules and regulations.

Third-Party Reimbursement Entities

Third-party payers will reimburse for physician services that are provided by a CNS if the services provided are within the scope of practice of the CNS and the payers' rules are adhered to. Unfortunately, the rules are often complex, difficult to find, and poorly understood. There are several categories of third-party payers that CNSs should be familiar with, including government entities such as Medicare, Medicaid, and Tricare; managed care organizations; and numerous commercial insurers. Each of these groups of payers has its own set of rules and criteria defining reimbursement policies, credentialing, and contracting and fee schedules. Medicaid and Medicare should be the starting point for your understanding of reimbursement and billing, as they have developed detailed policies and rules governing the reimbursement of providers that are used as the standard by other reimbursement entities. CNSs must possess sound knowledge of the structure, regulations, and reimbursement rules for each of the third-party entities with which they are involved. A clear understanding of the Medicare and Medicaid regulations pertaining to reimbursement will facilitate comprehension of other third-party-payer practices.

Medicare

Medicare was created as part of the Social Security Act of 1965 and is the federal health insurance program for the elderly and disabled. It is administered by the Centers for Medicare and Medicaid Services (CMS) of the United States Department of Health and Human Services. Previously known as the Healthcare Financing Administration (HCFA), CMS operates as an agent of the federal government and interprets Medicare laws and awards contracts on a state or regional level to manage billing and reimbursement programs (Frakes & Evans, 2006). These contracting agencies are named intermediary agencies for Medicare Part A or carriers for Part B. Medicare is administered locally by Medicare carrier agencies. There are two Medicare programs: Part A, or hospital insurance, covers inpatient hospital services and some home health care; Part B, which is also known as Supplemental Medical Insurance, covers the services of physicians and other selected providers like CNSs and NPs.

Medicaid

Medicaid is also a federal program administered by each state that provides coverage to low-income individuals and families, the elderly, and the disabled. Each state establishes its own Medicaid rules under federal guidelines. APNs can become Medicaid providers. Medicaid reimburses APNs at 70% to 100% of rates set for physicians.

How to Enroll in Medicare

Prior to enrolling in Medicare you must first obtain your National Provider Identifier (NPI). In the past the CNS would have had to complete applications to get a Unique Provider Identification Number (UPIN), a Medicare number, a Medicaid number, and then apply to each individual insurance company for a separate provider number! Exhausting and confusing to say the least. Now you just apply for your NPI number and you will use it forever for all billing transactions. You can apply for an NPI at http://nppes.cms.hhs.gov. The NPI replaces the previously used health care provider identifiers. A copy of the NPI notification letter you receive must then be included in the application to Medicare. To be eligible for reimbursement from Medicare, the CNS must first enroll in the program and be recognized as a provider by completing Form CMS-855I. This form can be found on the CMS Web site and downloaded at http://www.cms.hhs.gov/home/medicare.asp. The enrollment application is used to collect the required documentation to ensure you are qualified and eligible to enroll as a provider and includes professional licenses, the NPI notification letter, evidence of national certification, and evidence of a collaborative practice agreement with a physician. The definition of collaboration defers somewhat to state law in terms of how the exact collaborative arrangement is made. If you are practicing in a state that does not require a collaborative practice agreement, you only need to provide details about how you would communicate with a physician when an issue outside your scope of practice arises. The form must be completed in ink, preferably blue, signed, and mailed to the appropriate Medicare contractor that serves your state. A list of Medicare contractors can be found on the Web site as well (http://www.cms.hhs.gov/MedicareProviderSupEnroll/). The enrollment process takes approximately 60 days, sometimes longer.

Credentialing

Third-party payers vary in their requirements for credentialing for reimbursement, so it is necessary for CNSs to understand the specifics of each payer. In order to become a Medicare provider, a CNS must meet these requirements:

- Be a registered nurse who is currently licensed to practice in the state where he or she practices and be authorized to furnish the services of a CNS in accordance with state law
- Have a master's degree in a defined clinical area of nursing from an accredited educational institution, and
- Be certified as a CNS by a recognized national certification body that has established standards for CNSs (CMS Manual System, 2007). A list of approved national certifying bodies can be found on the CMS Web site.

Because Medicare has the most well-defined set of criteria and because other payers typically follow Medicare's lead, learning the basics of Medicare reimbursement is wise. The first step in the credentialing process is to determine which third-party payers are prevalent in your geographic area and in your practice. Next you should make a list of all of the health care plans, including the addresses, and telephone and fax numbers. Contact each entity by phone, requesting the name of the person responsible for credentialing and a copy of the credentialing application. You may have to request this in writing as well. Start a file on each health plan that you communicate with. The information required for each health care plan's credentialing is very similar to that required by Medicare. Be sure to make copies of everything sent out and keep accurate records for future reference. Be prepared to have to explain that you are a CNS and that you are an APN. You are often dealing with people who are more familiar with nurse practitioners and physician assistants and will not recognize the CNS.

Details of Reimbursement Regulations

The rules for reimbursement for physician services and the rules specific to APNs are complicated, vary from payer to payer, and are set according to state law. Numerous regulations govern health care reimbursement for all providers, and it is up to you to learn as much as possible. The more knowledgeable you are, the less likely you will be to make mistakes that could either cost you or your organization or result in denied charges. You cannot depend on your employer to take on this responsibility. The first requirement for reimbursement of medical services is that payment is made only for those services that are defined as *physician services* (Balanced Budget Act, 1997). When billing for a patient visit, codes are chosen that best represent the service provided. Two common sets of codes are CPT (Current Procedural Terminology) codes and ICD-9 (International Classification of Diseases) codes. These codes are organized into various categories and levels. Generally the more work performed—that is, the more complex the decision making—the higher the level of code selected within the appropriate category. CPT codes are 5-digit numeric codes developed by the American Medical Association to describe medical and diagnostic services, procedures, and the level of complexity of care (Baradell & Hanrahan, 2000). Updated each year, CPT codes attempt to provide a consistent, uniform language nationwide for communication among physicians, and other health care providers, patients, and third-payer parties. A CNS, as an APN, would submit a bill using the appropriate CPT code for the service provided. Thus you must be knowledgeable about the various CPT codes that exist. You can find accurate information in the CPT code manual, which is updated annually. You must select the CPT code that best represents the level of evaluation and management (E&M) service performed. For example, there are 5 CPT codes for an office visit for a new patient (99201–99205). You must choose the appropriate CPT code based on the level of E&M. The key components of the E&M service are the patient history, exam, and medical decision making and are defined by a set of documentation guidelines set forth by CMS. The more detailed or complex the visit, the higher the level of E&M code chosen and the higher the reimbursement. Documentation must support the level chosen and must meet the requirements for that level. Learning the required elements that must be performed in the history and physical exam, reflected in the decision making and documented, was one of the most difficult and lengthy processes for me to feel comfortable with. This included learning the type of medical decision making (straightforward, low, moderate, or high complexity), level of physical examination (detailed, problem focused, comprehensive), and determination of level of risk of complications (minimal, low, moderate, or high). E&M codes are universal and are used by Medicare, Medicaid, and other third-party payers. Again, there are numerous resources available to assist you in this process. Be prepared for a steep learning curve!

The other aspect of a reimbursement claim is the ICD-9 code. The ICD-9 coding system is used to communicate diseases, conditions, symptoms, and injuries. The original intent of these codes was to track mortality and epidemics. This code, also known as the diagnosis code, is used to provide the justification or medical necessity for a procedure or service provided. There are hundreds of ICD-9 codes that are used every day and can be found on the CMS Web site or in any hospital or physician billing department in the ICD-9 manual.

To review, for a service to qualify for Medicare reimbursement, several requirements must be met: The CNS must be legally authorized to perform the service; the service must be within the CNS's scope of practice; and some type of collaborative agreement with a physician must be in place. *Collaboration* is defined as a process in which the CNS works with a physician to deliver health care services within the scope of the practitioner's expertise, with medical direction and supervision as provided for in jointly developed guidelines or other mechanisms as provided by the law of the state in which the services are performed (Balanced Budget Act, 1997). When a CNS practices in a state that requires collaboration, Medicare requires nothing beyond what the state requires. If you are a CNS in a state without specific collaborative requirements for the CNS, you will be required to document your scope of practice and indicate the relationship you have with physicians to deal with any issues outside your scope of practice. Detailed instructions pertaining to services, qualifications, and conditions have been established and are outlined in the rules and regulations of the *Federal Register,* Volume 63, November 2, 1998, which can be found online under *Federal Register*.

Hospital-Employed CNSs

If you are a CNS employed by a hospital, one of the details you will have to clarify initially is whether your position falls under the global billing Medicare/Medicaid exempt category. If your position is classified as Medicare exempt, you will be unable to bill for any services. You should be able to determine this from discussion with someone in your human resources department. If you are not exempt and thus eligible to bill, you will also need to understand the rules surrounding the daily concurrent hospital billing done by the various providers.

Keeping Track of Productivity

When you begin to plan for billing for professional CNS services, it is extremely helpful to sit down with two people in your organization: your immediate supervisor and the person who will be submitting your billing statements. The latter is usually a certified coder. Developing a good working relationship with a coder can be of tremendous value as you embark on this learning expedition. The coder will have extensive knowledge of reimbursement, documentation requirements, and coding, and can be one of your best resources for questions. Networking with other CNSs in your organization who are already recognized Medicare providers can facilitate the process of learning and save you time and frustration as well. I also recommend that you discuss up front with your supervisor how the revenue generated by the services you provide will be handled. In some agreements, reimbursement for CNS services goes directly into the company and is considered a way of offsetting your salary. This seems, in my experience, to be the most common practice. You may want to negotiate some type of productivity bonus that you receive when a certain level of productivity is achieved. Another recommendation I have is to create some sort of tracking mechanism that will allow you to see how you are spending your time. For example, if your practice encompasses both hospital visits and clinic or office follow-up visits, you would want to be able to see where your time is spent and what level and types of services you are providing. In my own practice I received monthly printouts that showed the volume of hospital follow-up visits, admissions, discharges, consults, and procedures as well as the dollar amounts billed for each service. The amounts will vary depending on the level and type of service. The reimbursement allowed for each service will vary somewhat from year to year as well and is determined by the Physician Fee Schedule, which is updated annually. Reimbursement amount also depends on the individual third-party payer, with Medicare being one of the lowest payers. You will also want to know the average collection rate for services billed. This is another area where your billing person can come in handy. Depending on the type of practice you are in and the volume of "physician services" you provide, you may be amazed at the financial contribution you are making to an organization! Remember, in accordance with the Balanced Budget Act, CNS services are paid at 80% of the actual charge or 85% of the physician fee schedule amount, whichever is smaller. And that adds up! One word of caution: once an employer sees your revenue-generating potential, you will need to be careful not to allow exploitation of your services to generate more and more revenue by asking you to see more patients in a day. Don't allow your practice to become "assembly line" medicine. Remember, the essence of CNS practice is "clinical *nursing expertise* ..." (National Association of Clinical Nurse Specialists [NACNS], 2004). And although it is only those services delivered in the medical domain (i.e., physician services) that are currently reimbursed, a CNS has a larger responsibility for advancing the practice of *nursing* within nursing's autonomous scope (NACNS, 2004).

Conclusion

Although the rules and regulations of the reimbursement process can be overwhelming, it is important that the CNS have a good understanding of the regulations, terminology, and legalities surrounding reimbursement. Resources such as coding and billing seminars and conferences, independent study programs, continuing education programs, journal articles, and coding and billing experts are available and can provide valuable assistance. Sitting down with other CNSs who have already "mastered" the reimbursement puzzle can be invaluable. I say *mastered* in jest because in my experience it is an ongoing learning experience. Visit the government Web site for the Centers for Medicare and Medicaid Services to obtain firsthand up-to-date information. Your goal should be to understand current CPT and ICD-9 guidelines, requirements for accurate documentation of E&M codes, rules, regulations, and laws that govern you as a provider in your state to minimize your risk of fraudulent claims. Establish a process for timely, accurate reimbursement, thus reducing claim denials. You should be involved in every part of the process. Because of the dynamic nature of the reimbursement landscape, the CNS should be aware of these resources for billing and reimbursement and seek them out as opportunities for demonstrating the financial contributions of the CNS that will undoubtedly continue to grow. One last consideration for the CNS who bills is the increase in liability incurred. A well-intentioned provider can commit billing fraud if poorly informed. Even if your organization has a billing and coding department that actually prepares and submits the bill, you are accountable for knowing the rules and requirements for documentation for reimbursement. Prepare yourself by taking advantage of courses designed to help you learn and maintain current knowledge about billing rules and regulations. Additionally, you will need to ensure that you carry adequate liability insurance.

Billing and reimbursement issues may seem overwhelming at first, and are certainly challenging, but they can be fun and rewarding too! (See Table 20.1.)

20.1 The Language of Reimbursement

Acronym	Stands For	Definition
ICD-9	International Classification of Diseases, 9th edition	A system designed to standardize health care diagnoses for reimbursement purposes.
CPT Code	Current Procedural Terminology Code	A system designed by the American Medical Association to reimburse specific units of health care services.
OBRA	Ominbus Budget Reconciliation Act	Congressional acts that frequently have legislation related to health care.
MCO	Managed Care Organization	An entity that provides health care services and payment for the services provided. An umbrella term that can include a variety of organizations such as health maintenance organizations, provider-sponsored organizations, and physician hospital organizations.
RBRVS	Resource-Based-Relative-Value Scale	Complex federal regulations that rate health care activities for Medicare Part B reimbursement.
RVU	Relative Value Unit	A unit of health care that is specifically reimbursed according to rates set by CMS and vary according to level of care and geographical area.

(Continued)

20.1 The Language of Reimbursement *(Continued)*

Acronym	Stands For	Definition
DRGs	Diagnostic Related Groupings	A system of classification for inpatient hospital services based on diagnosis, age, sex, and presence of complications. It is used to identify costs of providing services and as a mechanism for predetermined reimbursement to a hospital based on the patient diagnosis.
CMS (previously HCFA)	Centers for Medicare and Medicaid Services (previously the Health Care Financing Agency)	Federal agency that determines rules and regulations for health care reimbursement policy.
FFS	Fee For Service	A reimbursement system where hospitals, physicians, and other providers are paid a specific amount for each service performed.
PPS	Prospective Payment System	A capitated reimbursement plan that provides payment based on designated amount per enrollee per year.
TRICARE (formerly known as CHAMPUS)	Civilian Health and Medical Program of the United States	Plan that provides health care to military personnel and their families.
FEHBP	Federal Employee Health Benefit Plan	Group insurance plan of federal employees and their dependents that recognizes APNs as providers.

References

Abood, S., & Keepnews, D. (2002). *Understanding payment for advanced practice nursing services Volume 2: Fraud and abuse*. Washington, DC: American Nurses Publishing.

Balanced Budget Act of 1997. (1997). United States Public Law 105-33: Subtitle F; Chapter 1- Services of Health Professionals; Subchapter B-Other Healthcare Professionals, Section 4511; August 5, 1997.

Baradell, J., & Hanrahan, N. (2000). CPT coding and Medicare reimbursement issues. *Clinical Nurse Specialist, 14*(6), 299–303.

CMS Manual System. (2007). Pub 100-08 Medicare Program Integrity Manual. Transmittal 219. Nurse Practitioner Services and Clinical Nurse Specialist Services Chapter 10, Section 12.4.5. Retrieved November 15, 2008, from http://www.cms.hhs.gov/Manuals/IOM/item detail.asp?filterType=none&filterByDID=99&sortByDID=1&sortOrder=ascending&itemID =CMSO19033&intNumPerPage=10

Frakes, M. A., & Evans, T. (2006). An overview of Medicare reimbursement regulations for advanced practice nurses. *Nursing Economics, 24*(2), 59–65.

National Association of Clinical Nurse Specialists (NACNS). (2004). *Statement on clinical nurse specialist practice and education* (2nd ed.). Harrisburg, PA: Author.

Richmond, T. S., Thompson, H. J., & Sullivan-Marx, E. M. (2000). Reimbursement for acute care nurse practitioner services. *American Journal of Critical Care, 9*(1), 52–61.

Zuzelo, P. R., Fallon, R., Lang, C., & Mount, L. (2004). Clinical nurse specialists' knowledge specific to Medicare structures and processes. *Clinical Nurse Specialist, 18*(4), 207–217.

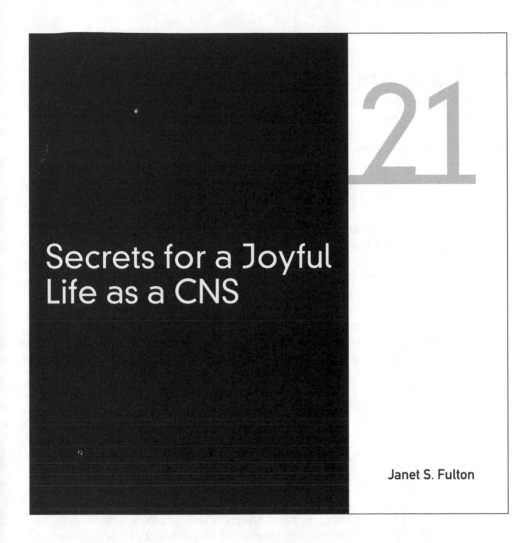

Secrets for a Joyful Life as a CNS

Janet S. Fulton

The purpose of this book is to offer some practical advice and considered perspective about the clinical nurse specialist (CNS) role for those beginning their career journey as CNSs. It is now my task in this final chapter to integrate the ideas and offer some sage advice. I decided to revisit some sage advice from Dr. Grayce Sills, Professor Emeritus, The Ohio State University, College of Nursing, as contained in her 1986 commencement address at Miami Valley School of Nursing in Dayton, Ohio. It was the last commencement for the hospital school of nursing, which had decided to close its doors in the face of increasing pressure for collegiate education for nurses. The address helped finalize an era and launch the future. A new CNS is in much the same position, leaving one period of a career behind while launching a new direction. Dr. Sills outlined 7 secrets for a joyful life in nursing. This chapter will revisit her 7 secrets, updated and reconsidered, for beginning a CNS career: life-long learning, collaboration, creative deviance, investment in the profession, families and communities, appreciation of difference, and humor.

Life-Long Learning

Life-long learning is a commitment to curiosity. Be curious and strive to ask good questions. Good questions are more important than correct answers. Could American ingenuity have landed a man on the moon and brought him back again unless someone first asked the question *can we go to the moon and back?* Forward direction is initiated by thoughtful, adventurous questions asked by really curious thinkers.

Knowledge serves to shape questions and provoke possibilities. Answers do not come from facts but rather from the intellectual work of asking questions, envisioning possibilities, and juxtaposing seemingly incongruent ideas. Knowledge is expanding at rates that no one could have predicted. Life-long learning has moved beyond responsibility for reading journals and attending professional conferences. While journals and conferences remain important, physical access to information is omnipresent electronically, thanks largely to the internet. Now life-long learning involves being a savvy evaluator of information.

Search for ideas in the most unlikely of places. The electronic information age requires only a mouse-click to find a new perspective and multiple worlds of ideas. Constantly ask questions about the reliability of information, but don't be so ready to dismiss misinformation, tall tales, and outright fabrications that circulate around the Web. Not all information may be reliable, but should it be summarily dismissed? Consider the implications.

Information from the Web can frame our perspective and inform our actions. An undergraduate student recently observed ketamine being used clinically and decided to write a paper about indications for use and nursing care of patients receiving the drug. When she searched the internet she found Web sites that provided instructions for abuse (how to have a *good K-trip*) and testimonials to the benefits of illegal use. This information was not what she intended to find; however, having found it, she decided to include a section in her paper about the drug's potential for abuse. If her search had been limited to professional journals, her information, and surely her perspective, would have been more limited.

Share your curiosities and innovations in presentations and publications. Dialogue with colleagues will help clarify ideas. Write. Nothing clarifies thinking like writing. Good writers are clear thinkers, or are clear thinkers good writers? Make time to write—schedule writing time and keep to it with the same dedication given to the seemingly endless list of committee meetings. Writing requires thinking, and thinking is learning. And once you've completed a piece of writing, publish it, so others can learn.

Collaboration

Life is a group project. Our very existence in a complex society requires collaboration. Health care settings are very complex systems where people's lives literally depend on the ability of the workers in the system to collaborate for common purpose. CNS course work includes content on collaboration in a multidisciplinary environment. This is fundamental and will become second nature for any CNS as time goes by. Invest early on in building collaborative relationships—it will return a thousand fold!

Think about collaboration as extending beyond the common notion of an *interdisciplinary health care team*. Consider the contributions of employees working in areas such as maintenance, supply services, housekeeping, parking, and the gift shop. Workers in these areas make critical contributions to the environment in which we practice. Flip the switch and the light goes on; fill the trashcan, and it is emptied; food trays are sterilized, drapes vacuumed, snow removed in winter. Consider what would happen if these workers were not part of the *environmental team*.

In her commencement address, Dr. Sills noted that in the mundane world of work, it is all too easy to get caught up in the invidious distinctions that divide us. It is good to remember the value that unites us—each of us desires the best possible end and the highest possible good for those we serve. Assume each person is working to the best of his/her ability. Commitment to teamwork means asking, "How can I help you?"

A hospital environment is a microcosm of society. It includes highly educated professionals with prestige and social privilege working alongside persons with minimal education and no professional credential. We serve a common purpose—work collaboratively, everyone included. The team is bigger than you think.

Collaborate within the professional community. Engage CNSs in other specialty areas and in other hospitals in projects and research. Projects start out with a burst of energy only to languish as work seems to drag and enthusiasm fades. Collaborating with others helps provide needed support and energy that will see the project to completion. Be a colleague, have a colleague.

Creative Deviance

Deviance is behavior that is sharply different from customary or traditional and is, in itself, value neutral. A CNS is, by design, a deviant nurse—someone who thinks differently and likewise acts differently. Embrace this difference; learn to wear it comfortably. Creative deviance is the source of innovation. Nurture your creativity by asking every day what can be done to improve quality, decrease cost, and enhance safety for patients and staff.

Creative deviance is contagious—be sure to infect the staff. Ask "I wonder if . . ." rhetorical questions in staff forums and committee meetings. Cultivate a climate of curiosity, and over time measure success by the number of new ideas that come from the staff. A staff nurse once asked my opinion about two methods for drawing blood from a central line. Rather than answer, I asked her what she considered to be the best method. She replied that in all her years of nursing, no one had ever asked her opinion. How sad, and yet what an opportunity! As a result of her initial inquiry, the procedure was changed. Creative deviance will flourish when staff are empowered.

Be kind and considerate, but persistent, as others will sometimes find your deviant thinking slightly irritating or perhaps downright annoying. Learn to read the rhythm of the situation, the ebb and flow of daily work demands, and group dynamics. But don't wait for consensus. While waiting for agreement, the window of opportunity may close. Consensus can also be a tyrant—demanding agreement in situations where difference should not only be allowed but encouraged.

Nursing has a convention of conformity, dating to our early history in military and religious traditions. Avoid the tyranny of consensus. Empower yourself to move ideas forward.

Investment in the Profession

As a nurse with a graduate degree, you are one of few in a profession of many. You are now an ambassador for the CNS role. Share your time and treasure by giving back. Join professional organizations and give back by serving in leadership or other positions. Give back by donating money to professional foundations that support nursing scholarships and research. Give back to your school. It's highly likely that somewhere in your career development you were helped along as a result of someone who gave back. It's your profession—invest in its future.

Families and Communities

Keep family first. Family is where your spirit resides, where you are nourished and loved. Family protects and defends. Family renews. Your health is intricately woven in the fabric of your family—your health is family health.

Remember that your family supported your education—sacrificed having your time and attention in exchange for classes and course work. Your family believes in you. Value your family's support by striving always to be the best that you can be.

Invest in your community. Communities are the harbingers of health values. Community investment occurs along a continuum. First, be informed. Read local publications and be aware of local issues that have health implications. Be informed about prevailing political sentiments, controversial issues, and the pros and cons associated with civic issues. Second, be present. Interact with others around common interests. Parents know that children's activities generate opportunities to be present—children's activities such as sporting events, music recitals, and school fundraising programs are ways to be present in a community. Other opportunities include civic associations and volunteering. Your presence as a parent/volunteer brings an advanced nursing perspective to your community. Third, influence others for a healthy community. Contribute to the community newspaper a health article in your area of specialty. Together with your local CNS network, create a list of specialty experts that local media can contact for commentary and informational contributions. Consider starting an "Ask a Nurse" column in the paper or for a radio talk show. Health and safety issues are embedded in many public policies. Support legislation that advances health. Meet with your local and state legislators; they need to know you and have you on their contact list when expert opinions are needed. Think about health and safety implications when communities deal with issues such as food labeling, bike helmet laws, immunization requirements, and other issues. As a leader in nursing, you can and should seek to influence the public welfare. Local politics is a perfect place to invest in the health of your community.

Appreciation of Difference

On a grand scale the world is shrinking every day—not literally in size, of course, but obstacles to human communication and interaction are disappearing. No longer is physical travel required to interact with others; the World Wide Web has made global "group projects" a norm. Like many of you are or will be, I'm a member of a project team that includes several different health care providers—nurses, physicians, dentists, dental hygienists, and pharmacists— from 10 different countries representing all 5 continents. It's a coming together around a topic of mutual interest for a common purpose. This kind of effort is the norm of the future. No more working in silos divided by profession, employment, country, or continent. Think globally.

Expanded cooperation between and among peoples of the world is pressing an even more urgent need to value human diversity. People tend to fear that which is different. Childhood experiences create our sense of familiar. The CNS should consider the extent to which personal experiences have prepared one for a diverse world. Fear of difference leads to suspicion, discrimination, petty meanness, and a tendency to develop forgone conclusions—all ways of thinking that will erode a CNS's ability to lead. Best to be amicable and approachable, because the ability to influence depends on others perceiving acceptance. Look for common ground and respect that which is different.

Humor

Take your work seriously and yourself lightly. Humor is found in recognizing oddities and inconsistencies in a situation, and the daily work of patient care in a complex system provides more than enough opportunity for humor. The ability to grin in the face of the bizarre and to laugh at incongruencies brings energy and renewal to both stiflingly boring tasks and epochs of human tragedy.

The well-known comedian George Carlin was a master at finding humor in inconsistencies. Here are some examples from his book *Brain Droppings* (Carlin, 1997):

- Shouldn't a complimentary beverage tell you what a fine person you are? (p. 89)
- In a hotel, why can't you use the house phone to phone your house? (p. 94)
- Every time you use the phrase *all my life* it has a different meaning. (p. 194)
- How is it possible to be seated on a standing committee? (p. 195)
- I put a dollar in one of those change machines. Nothing changed. (p. 197)

Things happen that are beyond our control, so look for humor and find joy. Every day comes with its own surprises.

Not every day will be full of joy, but each day can be an adventure in your personal pursuit of excellence. As you go forward in your new CNS role, make each day an adventure, stay curious, pursue excellence. Now I'll end this chapter with the same quote Dr. Sills used to end her address. Though dated in its publication, it is timeless in sentiment:

> A profession should make us more human, not less so; more alive, not less so; more dedicated, not less so; and we default on our professional birthright unless we can reach out to others and communicate this feeling of concern for the common bond between all of us. It is the food upon which your spirit feeds. It is the sustenance that helps motivate your patients to get well, or, rather, your fellow human to get well. You must give them this above all, and you must try even when they seem unable to accept it or profit by it. We fail others when we fail ourselves and when we succeed with ourselves we inevitably succeed with others. (Whitehouse, 1962)

References

Carlin, G. (1997). *Brain droppings.* New York: Hyperion.
Sills, G. M. (1986). *The quest for excellence: The joy of nursing.* Paper presented at the Eighty-eighth Commencement, Miami Valley Hospital School of Nursing, Miami, FL.
Whitehouse, F. A. (1962). The rational of nursing. *Rehabilitation Record, 3*(4), 12.